Energy SourceBook

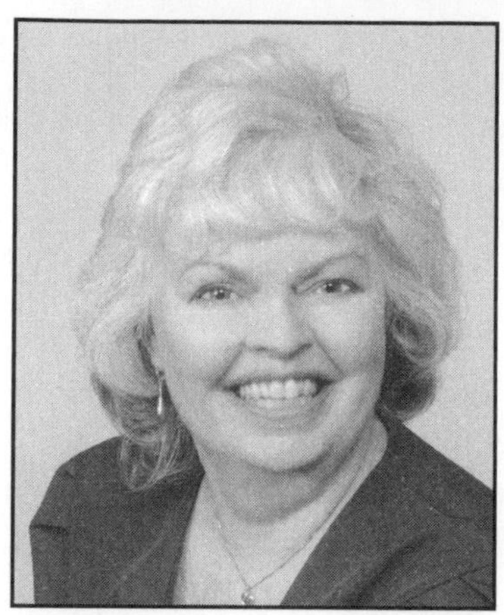

Dr. Jill Henry (North Carolina), Ed.D., PT, APP, is a leader in the metaphysical and alternative healing fields. Her mission is "to Explore, Facilitate, and Advance Well Being." With her academic background as a tenured Associate Professor of Physical Therapy and her dissertation research in Development and Learning for Transformation, Dr. Henry bridges the gap between traditional knowledge and the new paradigms of Energy Medicine and Self-Healing. She is a certified Associate Polarity Practitioner, a licensed Physical Therapist, a teacher, business owner, consultant, writer, speaker, and webmaster.

Dr. Henry has been presenting workshops in Meditation, Energy Healing, Paradigm Shifts, Adult Learning, and Self-Transformation for health-care professionals and academic faculties, business executives, and the general public for over twenty years. With her husband Charlie, she owns and operates a Web site, www.mountainvalleycenter.com, a well-being resource store, Mountain Valley Center, and the Otto Labyrinth Park in North Carolina's Smoky Mountains.

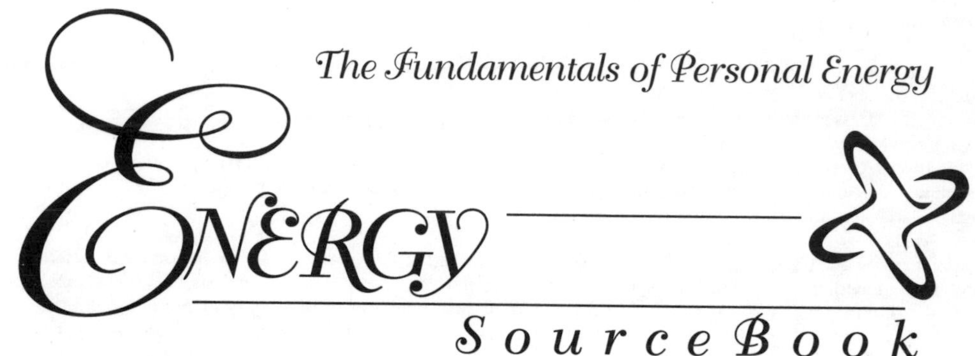

How to Balance, Increase, and Use It for Healing

Jill Henry, Ed.D.

2004
Llewellyn Publications
St. Paul, Minnesota 55164-0383, U.S.A.

First Edition
First Printing, 2004

Cover art © 2004 SuperStock
Cover design by Gavin Dayton Duffy

Library of Congress Cataloging-in-Publication Data
[to come]

Llewellyn Worldwide does not participate in, endorse, or have any authority or responsibility concerning private business transactions between our authors and the public.

All mail addressed to the author is forwarded but the publisher cannot, unless specifically instructed by the author, give out an address or phone number.

Any Internet references contained in this work are current at publication time, but the publisher cannot guarantee that a specific location will continue to be maintained. Please refer to the publisher's web site for links to authors' websites and other sources.

Disclaimer: The practices, techniques, and meditations described in this book should not be used as an alternative to professional medical treatment. This book does not attempt to give any medical diagnosis, treatment, prescription, or suggestion for medication in relation to any human disease, pain, injury, deformity, or physical condition.

The author and publisher of this book are not responsible in any manner whatsoever for any injury which may occur through following the instructions contained herein. It is recommended that before beginning any alternative healing practice you consult with your physician to determine whether you are medically, physically, and mentally fit to undertake the practice.

Llewellyn Publications
A Division of Llewellyn Worldwide, Ltd.
P.O. Box 64383, Dept. 0-7387-0529-2
St. Paul, MN 55164-0383, U.S.A.
www.llewellyn.com

Printed in the United States of America

Dedicated to the Well Being of all of us
from individuals to communities to the world.
May all beings be well.

Contents

Section Three

Polarity Energy, the Five Elements, and You

Section Four

Feng Shui: The Energy of Your Environment

References and Resources

List of Tables

Introduction

In 1988, working on my dissertation in Adult Education at the University of Georgia, I developed a model of Development and Learning for Transformation. This model was all theory—what I believed could and should happen as we grow and change.

During the last sixteen years, I have been learning and experiencing the "how-to's" of the original model—the real work, and play, of growing and changing as adults.

I offer this book as an integration of theory and practical experience. Inside you will find tools, techniques, and practices to bring well-being into your life. You will need no fancy equipment, no additional purchases, to discover "Well Being"—just your own mind. I will show you how to travel beyond a limited, personal state of consciousness into the realms of Well Being and self-realization. There, the small ego self releases to the Universal Self and the path of Well Being becomes clear.

The Meaning of Well Being

The dictionary defines "well" in the following manner: "to rise to the surface and flow forth; to pour from the depths; healthy, prosperous; in a satisfactory state; without doubt or question; with skill or aptitude; expertly, naturally; and being a cause for thankfulness." "Being" is defined as: "existence, life, the essence and personality of a living thing."

Combining these two words, and their definitions, into one reveals a new, transformed person. A "Well Being" is a person whose essence has risen from the depths to the surface and now flows naturally forth in health and prosperity, to live life with skill and thankfulness. The energy of Well Being is capable of transforming fear into love, illness into wellness, isolation into unity, and work into calling. Well Being enables you, and me, to cope with and effect change in our lives, and to improve the quality of not only our own lives, but also the lives of people around us.

Accessing the Energy of Well Being

A state of Well Being is developed by first understanding that a flow of energy underlies all physical and mental processes. Beneath the apparent physical and mechanical surface is a holistic, organismic flow of pure energy. This energy is constantly being directed by our thoughts, emotions, and feelings. To access this energy, to experience it firsthand, requires certain knowledge and skills. This book is a practical guide to developing those skills.

I have divided the book into four major sections:

Using Relaxation and Meditation as Tools for Change
Exploring the Energy of the Chakras
Polarity, the Five Elements, and You
Feng Shui—The Energy of Your Environment

Each section stands alone as a path to well-being. In addition, each chapter in each section stands alone. Pick a chapter, read the theory, and try the suggested practices. The chapters are short, so that you may spend less time reading and more time *doing*. It is only when you are experiencing that you feel the flow of energy. It is by feeling that flow that a higher state of Well Being is attained. So feel the flow and enjoy the experience!

You may journey through this book chapter by chapter, or you may simply pick a chapter at random, read the theory, and practice the exercises. There are no rules, only understanding and experience. Many blessings on your journey to Well Being.

— Dr. Jill Newman Henry

Acknowledgments

Without the spiritual energy, guidance, and support of my husband, Charlie Henry, this book would have not been written. Over twenty years ago, we began a spiritual path together. That path has taken us from professors in Physical Therapy at the Medical College of Georgia to entrepreneurs in the Western North Carolina Mountains. Along this path we have developed trust in the guidance of the unseen Universe and are learning together to replace fear with faith and love. Thank you, Charlie, for being with me on this journey.

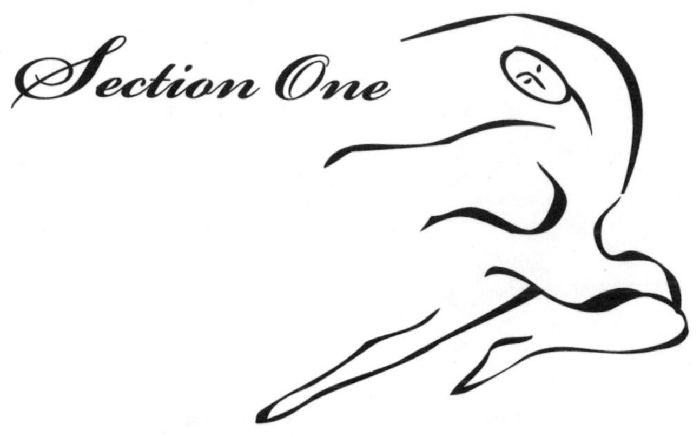

Using Relaxation and Meditation as Tools for Change

This section guides you through a developmental sequence of activities, from basic relaxation skills to deep meditative practices.

You may choose to follow in sequence, or skip directly to the chapter that interests you most at this time. You can always return to previous chapters. As in every chapter in this book, the most important thing is to decide to do something with the information presented. Even if you only set aside ten minutes each day to practice relaxation or meditation, you will experience the benefits.

While working through this section, keep in mind that in our Western culture, practicing relaxation and meditation is often viewed as "wasting time." We have learned to keep busy doing things in the external world and sometimes may be seen as being selfish when we attend to our own inner worlds. Yet it is our inner worlds that manifest into the outer. The more peaceful, happy, and confident you feel inside, the more you will have experiences of these in the outer world. Life truly is an "inside job."

One

Changing World

Change has always been a part of life, but never before has it appeared so rapidly, with such pervasive effects. The changes caused by the events of September 11, 2001, have left their mark in all aspects of society. The speed of change in the scientific, political, and technological worlds has altered the basic meaning of work, leisure, relationships, health, distance, and time. Threat of obsolescence in the workplace, psychological uncertainty and anxiety over how to adapt to change, are part of everyday life. In addition, change is occurring in our basic beliefs about knowledge and knowing. Vaughan (1986) describes three types of knowledge: *empirical,* obtained by direct perception through the senses; *rational,* obtained through intellectual reasoning and cognition; and *transcendental* obtained through contemplation and meditation. During the current industrial and technological age, the majority of society has used perception and cognition exclusively as sources of knowledge.

Capra (1982) and Ferguson (1980) describe a paradigm shift away from the exclusive use of perception and cognition, toward an understanding of reality and living through contemplation of a universal wholeness or interconnectedness. Physicists, attempting to explain quantum theory through perception and cognition, discovered they could not. Their attempts to find a unified theory of physics resulted in the discovery of unity, harmony, and oneness, concepts that cannot be explained by rational thinking. "The universe is no longer seen as a machine, made up of a multitude of objects, but has to be pictured as one indivisible, dynamic whole, whose parts are essentially interrelated and can be understood only as patterns of a cosmic process" (Capra, 1982, p. 78). Subatomic particles are not material "things" but potentials, tendencies, or probabilities that exist only as interconnections between aspects of the whole. There is a dynamic flow to the universe and this flow is affected by everything in it. In the new physics, the observer affects the observed because both are part of the same One.

Philosophically, the implications of the new physics are "that the basic structures of the material world are determined, ultimately, by the way we look at this world; that the observed patterns of matter are reflections of patterns of mind" (Capra, 1982, p. 93). These patterns of mind are discovered through internal contemplation, using techniques such as relaxation and meditation, not external viewing and judging.

Coping Strategies for Stress and Change

There are many strategies for coping with our changing world. Some are better than others. The best ones direct us inward as we develop relaxation and meditation. This section is designed to explore in depth these techniques. However, in order to be complete, we will briefly review all coping strategies in this first chapter.

Indirect Coping Strategies

Strategy 1: Drug and Alcohol Abuse. This strategy is not highly recommended, but is often used. Drugs and alcohol keep our anxieties below the threshold of awareness. If we are not aware of inner tension, then we do not have to do anything about it. That is, we do not have to grow and change.

Strategy 2: Psycho-physiological Illness. Illness represents a legitimate "time out." It is a way to enter meditative states without guilt. After all, when we are ill, we have to stay in bed; we are encouraged to relax and "get well." Now, I am not saying that anyone, anywhere, consciously chooses to become ill, or to acquire a disease, or to have an accident. I am saying that deep down in the mass consciousness, illness does represent a way out of our current stress. It substitutes a new stress for the old stress that "made" us sick in the first place, and therefore helps us change. It is no coincidence that the word disease can be shown as "dis-ease," or "lack of ease" in the body/mind. Assuming we do not wish to use this strategy for coping, let us move on.

Strategy 3: Defense Mechanism. Defense mechanisms are attempts to get rid of stress by placing stress outside us. Rationalization allows us to not feel responsible, and therefore not guilty (of whatever it is that we think we "should" feel guilty about). When we project blame, we are literally trying to throw our stress out of us. Unfortunately, our stress is actually tied to us like a rubber ball, which comes bouncing back! Stirring up conflict is another defense mechanism often used. When we "stir the pot," we hope to get the stress away from us so fast that none of it will "stick." Again, these are perhaps not the best ways of coping.

Strategy 4: Escape and Avoidance. We try to escape or avoid stress by: leaving early, avoiding peers, increasing isolation, long lunch breaks, spending more time with paperwork, spending time in front of the TV or computer . . . the list goes on and on. I imagine you can think of several of your favorite ways to avoid stress right now!

Direct Coping Strategies

Strategy 1: Relaxation Techniques. Relaxation techniques are used as a principle means of coping when the environment is changing rapidly. They are used to "relearn" how to respond to stressful situations and include formal techniques like progressive relaxation, hypnotic induction, sensory awareness, meditation, autogenic training, biofeedback, visualization and imagery, yoga, Tai Chi and Chi Gong and many more. We will be exploring many of these techniques in depth in the following chapters.

Strategy 2: Exercise. Exercise is important to both mind and body. To gain the most benefit from exercise, it must be both regular and pleasurable. If your exercise is "stressing you out," then it is time to learn the art of relaxation and apply it to your daily routines. In future chapters we will look at the application of mindfulness to exercise.

Strategy 3: Diet. Ayurvedic medicine describes foods based on the Doshas, or body/mind types, that influence our minds, emotions, and general state of Well Being. The following is a brief outline of foods you may use to relax.

To calm worry, fear, anxiety . . .

- Favor foods that are sweet, sour and salty.
- Reduce your intake of foods that are pungent, bitter, and astringent.

To cool off from anger or frustration . . .

- Favor foods that are sweet, bitter, and astringent.
- Reduce your intake of pungent, sour, salty foods.

To stimulate and prevent procrastination, and resistance to change . . .

- Favor foods that are astringent, pungent, bitter.
- Reduce your intake of sweet, sour, and salty foods.

Examples of Foods

Sweet: sugar, milk, butter, rice, breads, pasta

Salty: sea salt

Sour: yogurt, lemon, cheese, vinegar

Pungent: spicy foods, peppers, ginger

Bitter: spinach, green leafy vegetables

Astringent: beans, lentils, honey

Strategy 4. Changing Oneself. This involves a shift of perspective or paradigm shift about the nature of your stress and problems. The word paradigm stems from the Greek word *paradeigma* or "pattern." A paradigm is a scheme for understanding and explaining certain aspects of reality. Paradigms represent the thoughts, values, and assumptions that underlie a culture or a society. A paradigm shift involves a new way of thinking about an old problem and the emergence of a new level of consciousness concerning the attributions one makes about the causes of and solutions to problems. Relaxation and meditation provide valuable tools for paradigm shifts, allowing us to let go and take control of our lives and our world in more positive and healthy ways.

Choosing a Strategy

This book is filled with successful strategies for not only coping with, but also effecting change in your life. To begin, try one of the following quick ways to de-stress and change negative energy into Well Being.

The Four-Count

Count silently to four while you inhale, and hold for four counts. Count silently to four while you exhale, then hold for four counts. Repeat for up to five minutes.

The Ten-Count

Count to ten! But do it so you are totally aware of each breath you count. If you "forget" to feel a breath, start over and try again.

Bodybreath

Inhale through your fingertips, up your arms and into shoulders and head. Exhale down your neck, abdomen, legs and out to your toes.

Peacebreath

Inhale while visualizing peace in-filling your body (head to toes) . . . pause, and then exhale while visualizing tension leaving body (toes to head).

Groaning to Relax

For five minutes, give yourself and those around you permission to loudly groan away the stresses that have been building during the day.

Laughing to Relax

Take a laughter break—for five minutes, just laugh!

Progressive Relaxation

Tighten, then relax, each major muscle group in your body. Begin at the feet and work up toward your head (toes, ankles, calves, knees, thighs, buttocks, stomach, back, hands, wrists, elbows, shoulders, neck, head, face).

Autogenic Training

Mentally breath into each body part listed above, feeling warmth and relaxation begin to flow in each area.

Petting Animals

Find a dog, cat, or other pet—simply sit down and pet them!

Self-Imagery

In your mind, recreate a relaxing place you have experienced in the past. Return to that place and "live" there for a few seconds or minutes.

Guided Imagery

Recorded tapes and CDs usually take the listener to a special place, a waterfall, mountain, meadow, ocean . . . and guide the listener through a series of releasing and healing images.

Music

The most relaxing music contains sounds with a natural rhythm and no melody. The sound is cyclical and repeated.

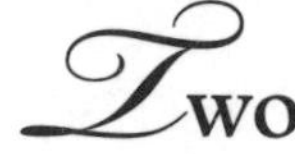

Two

Stress or Relaxation?

Many people believe that stress is entirely dependent upon their life situations. Some people simply have more stressful lives than others and, to an extent, that is true. It is more stressful when living with too many responsibilities, being constantly dissatisfied, or having chronic worries. These three factors are influenced by our patterns of behavior and play a great part in our general level of stress or relaxation.

Relaxation is a choice we can make as we go along life's paths. We must, however, know* how *and* what *to choose.

Stress Due to Too Many Responsibilities

You are feeling stress due to excessive responsibilities when:

- You find yourself with not enough time to complete your work.
- You often become confused and cannot think clearly because too many things are happening at once.
- You become depressed considering all the things that you need to do.
- You skip meals so you can get your work done.

Stress Due to Dissatisfaction

Your stress is coming from dissatisfaction when:

- You get upset when someone in front of you drives too slowly.
- It bothers you when your plans depend upon the actions of others.
- You become anxious when your plans don't flow smoothly.
- You hate to have your activities and plans disturbed by anything or anyone.

Stress Due to Worry

Your stress is due to chronic worry when:

- You tend to imagine all the worst possible things that could happen to you as a result of whatever "crisis" you are in.
- You re-live in your mind the crisis over and over again, even though it may be over and resolved.
- You are able to picture the crisis clearly in your mind weeks after it is over and done with.
- You can feel your heart pound in your chest, or your muscles tense up.
- You have so many thoughts in your head that you actually have difficulty thinking.

Our initial attitude toward a life event determines our stress—not the event itself. To one person, a roller coaster ride is stressful; to another, it is a form of relaxation. We have learned to interpret events as stressful or relaxing from our families and friends. For example, to my mother, going on a car trip was stressful. "What if the brakes failed? What if we ran out of gas? What if we blew out a tire? . . ." For years after leaving home, I developed high levels of stress whenever I thought of driving away. Then two events occurred. I bought a car I loved and I took a position at a university that required a lot of car trips. Between enjoying driving my new car, and looking forward to meeting new people and seeing new places expense-paid, I relearned to enjoy trips by car.

How many of the following stress attitudes have you inherited?

- Waiting in lines is always stressful.
- If something takes too long, it's only natural to become upset.
- It is all right to lose your temper under stress—everyone does it.
- It's not worth doing anything if I'm not going to win!
- It's better to do two or three things at once, like eating while working or planning while driving or bathing. That way, things get done!
- You should feel guilty when you are not actively working on something.

We can relearn only by changing our perceptions about our life and our world. Perceptions are our way of "making meaning," and are based upon our beliefs about others and ourselves. Changing beliefs and perceptions is not easy, but it can be done. In the coming chapters, we will take concrete steps to release old perceptions and gently acquire new ones. For now it is enough to state that if our perceptions are nonloving, then we will experience stress. If our perceptions are loving, then relaxation is sure to follow—*no matter what the life event.*

Perceptions and Making Meaning

The present moment is our point of personal power. It is where we perceive and make meaning. A positive past makes it easy to see the future with optimism. A negative past tends to promote a pessimistic future. *But* we have the ability to choose in the present moment, regardless of our past. Read these definitions:

Pessimism (n.) The tendency to exaggerate in thought the evils of life.

Pessimist (n.) One who looks on the worst side of everything.

Optimism (n.) The doctrine that all is for the best; the habit of looking at the brighter side of life.

Optimist (n.) One who believes that things are all right and takes a cheerful and hopeful view of life.

What Do You Choose Right Now?

In the present moment, you have the power to choose an optimistic or pessimistic future. The beauty of your choice is that when you choose for optimism, you create it in the present and the present becomes the past of the next moment. Moment by moment we can choose to create faith, love, and joy. Awesome, isn't it?

Once we perceive an event to be nonloving, we automatically generate strong, negative emotions. Once we perceive an event to be loving, we generate calm, positive emotions. Traditional stress management is devoted to managing negativity after it has occurred. Our approach is to prevent its occurrence as much as possible. We will not neglect stress management, but we will focus on relaxation attainment.

Once strong emotions have developed, physical effects occur. Strong negative emotions such as anger, hurt, anxiousness, fear, insecurity, resentfulness, and general unhappiness can manifest as chronic muscle tension, increased intestinal disturbances, increased nervous system activity, increased metabolic demands, increased heart rate, high blood pressure, and decreased immunity—to name just a few! Strong positive emotions such as calmness, happiness, friendliness, serenity, compassion, joy and peace will manifest as relaxed muscles, free flow of circulation, normal heart rate and rhythm, normal blood pressure, increased functioning of the immune system, and natural body balance and flow.

The choice of stress or relaxation is up to you. The choice lies at the level of perception. (See Table 1 at right.) Life events occur. How you perceive them takes you automatically down the path of stress or relaxation. No one can tell you to "relax" once the perception has generated a nonloving emotion and its corresponding physical effects. You must then take time to "work out" of them and return to a state of loving. The secret to relaxation has to do with staying in the present moment, and letting a peaceful present generate a peaceful future. That is the point of power and the subject of our next chapter.

Stress		Relaxation
Negative, judgmental.	**Life Situations**	Positive, accepting.
Non-loving interpretations of others and our world result in stress.	**Perceptions** **making meaning (perceptions can be changed)**	Loving interpretations of others and our world result in relaxation.
Stress producing emotions are strong and negative: Anger, fear, hurt, anxiety, insecurity, unhappiness, resentfulness . . .	**Emotions**	Relaxation producing emotions are comforting and positive: Calmness, happiness, friendliness, joy, compassion, wonder . . .
Stress manifests as: Chronic muscle tension, increased intestinal disturbances, increased nervous system activity, increased metabolic demands, increased heart rate, high blood pressure, and decreased immunity.	**Physical Effects**	Relaxation manifests as: Relaxed muscles, free flow of circulation, normal heart rate and rhythm, normal blood pressure, increased functioning of the immune system, and natural body balance and flow.
"Dis-ease" occurring as illness, worry and fear.	**Outcome**	Ease occurring as health, happiness, and well-being.

TABLE 1. STRESS OR RELAXATION?

Three

Thought Patterns: Worry or Affirm?

The present moment is the only one with which we have to work. The problem is we have crowded it with our past memories and future longings. How many times have you relived past conversations, reviewing things you "should" have said or done. When this occurs, you are mentally bringing those past experiences into your present moment. You are inviting them into your home, your bed, just as if they were really present. And then there is the future, full of worry, doubt, and fear. Of course, the past may have good memories that are fun to relive, and the future may contain joyous expectations of good things to come. But they are still past and future, and keep you from living now, fully in the present.

Consider your first response to the following questions:

When I get up in the morning, I most often think about ________________.

During the day, I typically think about________________________________.

During the evening, I often think about ____________________________.

Just before falling asleep, I think of ______________________________.

On vacation, I most often think about ____________________________.

If you are like most people, you answered the questions like this:

When I get up in the morning, I most often think about *what I'm going to do, have to do, want to do today.*

During the day, I typically think about *what I should have done and what I need to do.*

During the evening, I often think about *what I didn't do that I wanted to do.*

Just before falling asleep, I think of *what I need to do tomorrow and what I did today.*

On vacation, I most often think about *nothing, I just took it all in, I didn't think about anything, I just was . . .*

	Past	Present	Future
Pattern A	☑	☒	☒
"Living in the past" *What might have been* *What happened when . . .* *What was done to me*			
Pattern B	☒	☒	☑
"Living in the future" *What might happen if . . .* *What I want/don't want to happen*			
Pattern C	☑	☒	☑
"State of confusion" *Bouncing between loss/guilt vs. anticipation/fear*			
Pattern D	☒	☑	☒
"Living in the present moment" *The only point of action and personal power*			

TABLE 2. TYPICAL PATTERNS OF THOUGHT

Our minds are constantly buzzing between past thoughts and future thoughts. It seems that it is only when we go on vacation that we can concentrate on the present—on the mountains or ocean or sunset. Four typical thought patterns are shown in Table 2 at left. Can you find yourself?

Let's look at a prime example of living in the future—living with *worry*. Many of us learned to worry from our parents and have developed it into a fine art. "What if I fail? What if she/he leaves me? What if I get sick? What if I will not have enough money?" etc. Symptoms of worry include restlessness and feeling edgy, easy fatigability, concentration difficulties, irritability, muscle tensions and aches and restless sleep. I saw a TV commercial recently advertising a pill you can take to suppress worry. Pills are nice for a quick fix, but worry, like all past or future thoughts, is a symptom of a deeper problem—the inability to control our own minds. Our thoughts are there, thousands and thousands of them. They are triggered by what we see, what we hear, what we smell, what we do. The purpose of this section is to learn techniques to gain control of our mind, to choose new thoughts and to explore new ways of viewing the world. The first technique we will learn right now is affirmations.

We are affirming all the time. Every thought accompanied by belief or expectation is an affirmation. The problem is that most of the time we affirm exactly what we do not want. "I feel sick; I don't have enough money; I never get any rest; I don't like . . . I don't have . . . etc." Recognize any of those affirmations? What keeps our affirmations from being in the present moment is that we are bringing our *past* beliefs into the equation. Those past beliefs are guiding our *future* by their presence in our *now*. Since at this time we believe we have to think something, why not think about what we want to have in the future *now?* That's the secret of affirmations. To affirm in the present what appears to be not there with the belief that it is there, so it will be there! Sounds crazy—but with the right tools, affirmations can work for you. You are using them all the time; why not change the negative ones to positives and see the results for yourself?

One of the most famous affirmations came from a French physician in the nineteenth century, Dr. Coué. He was treating patients using mostly the same techniques as his peers, but his patients kept getting better, faster. His peers became curious about what he was doing that they were not. Finally they asked him. Dr. Coué said, "It's simple. All I do is tell my patients to repeat the following sentence as often as they can throughout their waking moments. If they do, they get better!" The famous sentence is, *"Every day, in every way, I am getting better and better."* Said with conviction and belief, this is a powerful statement, one that can make the difference between sickness and healing. There is one caveat however. If, for every time I affirm, "Every day, in every way, my life is better and better." I have fifty or a hundred affirmations such as *"But I don't feel good now . . . I'm tired . . . I'm broke . . . I'm lonely . . . I'm bored . . . I'm . . ."* My negative affirmations tend to cancel out the positive. In addition, we often put more energy and belief into the negative than the positive.

One technique I have used for uncovering the negative is inspired by our friend Barrie Konicov of Potentials Unlimited and detailed in his *Will Power* tape. Another excellent source for turning *wants* into reality is the book *Excuse Me, Your Life is Waiting* by Lynn Grabhorn.

To develop affirmations that work, take out a piece of paper and draw a line from top to bottom, down the middle of the paper. On the left side of the paper write: I WANT, then write down what you want to have in your life that you do not already have. Now, for each "I want" on the left side of the paper, on the right side, write down all the negative thoughts that come to mind telling you why what you want isn't possible. After each negative thought, say, "Thank You." You are thanking the hidden thought for coming into the light of your consciousness and releasing it!

Now do the same exercise using I CAN on the left side of the paper and continuing to list your hidden thoughts on the right side (see examples at right).

Now change your "can" statement into a "will" statement, by writing next to it: "and prove everyone wrong." Now the statement, "and prove everybody wrong" sounds a bit negative. However, often what is blocking your achievement is a deep, underlying commitment to meet everyone's expectations of you. "The rich get richer while the poor get poorer" is a good example of a cultural expectation. If you are not rich (or loved, or healthy, or whatever you are working on), perhaps it is because of a deeper need to be as others see you. Try writing this statement with a few affirmations and notice how you feel.

I Want . . .	**But . . .**
To have lots and lots of money to pay off all my bills and have money to share with others . . .	. . . It's impossible for me. *Thank you!* . . . Only rich people have money and I'm poor. *Thank you!* . . . Money doesn't grow on trees. *Thank you!* . . . If I haven't earned it now, I never will. *Thank you!* . . . I'm not good enough to earn enough. *Thank you!* *Keep writing until nothing else comes to the surface!*

I Can . . .	**But I Can't Because . . .**
Have lots and lots of money to pay off all my bills and have money to share with others . . .	. . . I'd have to work too hard. *Thank you!* . . . I don't have the right job. *Thank you!* . . . I can't see how I'm ever going to have money. *Thank you!* . . . I can't see an end to my bills. *Thank you!* *Keep writing until nothing else comes to the surface!*

I will have lots and lots of money and pay off all my bills and have money to share with others and prove everybody wrong!

I will heal my body and recover from this illness and prove everybody wrong!

I will find my soulmate and prove everybody wrong!

Finally, write your want/can/will into an affirmation in the present tense.

I am rich. I have money coming to me today in great quantities of abundance!

I am healthy now. I feel great!

If you have gone through the process successfully (and it may take several times to do so), your final affirmation will carry with it a feeling of power and belief. Now use this affirmation constantly. Say it, sing it, write it, read it. Tune your subconscious mind to making it a habit. The affirmation becomes your first thought upon waking and your last thought upon going to sleep, and with infinite patience, watch it appear in your life!

There is an old song whose lyrics go: "Accentuate the positive, eliminate the negative, latch on to the affirmative, and don't mess with Mr. In-Between." That song is the secret of affirmations, of creating positive, present thoughts and feelings that will result in positive, wonderful future present moments. Good luck and good affirming!

Four

Techniques to Relax the Body

Though the body is not separate from the mind, often we need to calm the body before we can calm the mind. The following are some general considerations for self-help techniques to relax your body.

Did You Know That . . . ?

- Chronic muscle tension works against peak performance, wastes energy, and causes injury and anxiety in athletes.
- Deep, relaxed, diaphragmatic breathing (abdominal breathing) increases the production of endorphins, the body's own morphine-like painkilling substances.
- Each year doctors write 50 million prescriptions for tranquilizers—yet they do not get at the cause of anxiety.

The following are techniques that help relax the body. They are all easy to do! The difficult part is doing them consistently. Any one of the following, when done daily for prevention, will result in marked change from body "dis-ease" to body ease. When the techniques are performed only as "emergency measures" they are less effective.

Breathing Techniques

Breathing techniques are used to quickly relax the body. When the breath slows down, messages are sent to the adrenal system that "all is well," thus depressing the stress "fight or flight" response. Breathing with awareness can instantly relax body and mind.

Technique

- Inhale, imagining your breath flowing through your fingertips, up the arms into the shoulders, then exhale down the trunk, into abdomen and legs and leisurely out the toes.
- Place your hands on your abdomen, feel it rise and fall as you breathe deep into your belly. Now count to three during each inhale, count three while hold your breath, and count three during each exhale, and three more while holding the breath. Allow the body to relax deeper and deeper.
- Try inhaling for six seconds and exhaling for seven seconds, for two minutes. Hint—to count, mentally say a number, then a three-syllable word to equal one second, i.e., "One el-e-phant, two el-e-phant . . ."
- To balance yin/yang (male/female, right side/left side) energy, breathe in this method taught in Kyria Yoga schools of study. Place your hand over your nose, with thumb on one nostril, index finger on the bridge of your nose, and your middle finger gently on the other nostril. Now close one nostril with your thumb, and breathe gently and deeply in and out through the other nostril. After a minute or so, reverse and close the other nostril and breathe in and out through the nostril under your thumb. Let the energy move until it feels complete. Now, try alternate breathing. Close one nostril with your thumb and breathe in through the other. Reverse on the exhale by opening the thumb nostril and closing the middle-finger side. Now open the thumb nostril and inhale. Exhale through the other nostril. With practice, you will soon find a soothing rhythm to your breath as you balance your energies through alternate nostril breathing.

Progressive Relaxation

"Progressive Relaxation" was coined by Dr. Edmund Jacobson, who equated mental stress with muscle tension that, in turn, contributed to more mental stress. He described the tense-mind, tense-muscle cycle and prescribed a technique to break the cycle and induce relaxation.

Technique

- Lie down, close your eyes and place your attention on your toes.
- Bend your toes and tighten, tighten, tighten, Hold, now relax. Repeat two or three times until you become aware of the feeling or relaxation in your toes.
- Progress through every body part: toes, ankles, calves, knees, thighs, hips, buttocks, abdomen, chest, back, shoulders, arms, elbows, wrists, hands, neck, face, mouth, eyes, scalp.
- Return to any body part that still feels tense, tighten and relax.
- Lie still and allow relaxation to flow through your body.

Autogenic Training

"Autogenic Training" is a mental variation of Progressive Relaxation. Instead of actually moving muscles, you "move energy" in your mind. By directing energy to various body parts, you allow feelings of warmth and relaxation to occur. In one study, a patient was placed on a circular platform perfectly balanced upon a center point. Simply by thinking about a body part, the platform moved. When the patient thought about his head, the platform tilted down at the head. The same was true when thinking about all other body parts—feet, arms, etc. This simple study validated the power of simply directing thoughts and energy to areas of our body that require relaxation.

Technique

- Imagine a ball of light and warmth, sparkling just above the top of your head.
- Bring this ball of energy and light down into your head and feel it massaging all the cells and tissues in your brain, scalp, and face with its healing light.
- Progress the ball down through the head, face, neck, shoulders, arms, hands, chest, abdomen, pelvis, back, hips, thighs, knees, ankles, and feet.
- Allow the energy to circulate through your whole body.
- Feel the light shining away all darkness.
- Allow the light to move through the pores of your skin, surrounding you in a halo of light.
- Gradually open your eyes and move around.

Relaxercise

"Relaxercise" is a series of ten exercises based upon the work of Dr. Moshe Feldenkrais's *Awareness Through Movement.* Each exercise consists of gentle, slow, repeated movements of different body parts within a pain-free range of motion. These gentle, slow movements assist the body in releasing stored tension and regaining comfortable movement. The following provides a general idea of the type of exercise involved. Study with a certified Feldenkrais practitioner for the full program and exercise sequences.

Technique

- Sit upright in a straight chair with your back against the chair-back.
- Slowly turn your upper trunk, neck, and shoulders to the left. Notice how far you can go comfortably by noting a spot on the wall behind you.
- Repeat this motion slowly, six to ten times.

- Now turn to the left while keeping your head straight in front of you. Repeat six to ten times.
- Now turn to the left with your trunk and head, while keeping your eyes looking straight in front of you. Repeat six to ten times.
- Now turn trunk, head, and eyes to left. Can you see any farther behind you?
- Repeat the above while turning to the right.

Yoga

Yoga forms of exercise are remarkable for releasing tension and reducing stress. In yoga you assume different postures while placing gentle stretches on different body areas. Yoga postures are precise and have been used for centuries to relieve physical and mental "dis-ease," as well as a path to higher spiritual understanding. The best way to learn yoga is to find a good teacher in your area and take a class. Books and videotapes are available when you cannot find a teacher. The following is one example of thousands.

Technique

- Lie on the floor on your stomach. Place your hands next to your shoulders and gently lift up, arching your back and allowing a stretch to occur in the stomach and chest area.
- Now push back and rest your buttocks on your heals, with toes stretched forward and stretch your arms out in front of you on the floor.
- Lift up into a "hands and knees" position, then continue on down until you are once again lying on the floor.
- Release toes backward and relax.
- Repeat five to ten times, slowing, and enjoying the stretch.

Tai Chi, Chi Gong

Tai Chi and Chi Gong are forms of relaxation experienced by performing simple, commonplace movements in very specific ways. They are designed to facilitate the flow of life energy, Chi, and release blocks. They require instruction, preferably from a master. I studied with Luke Chan, a Chinese master of Chi Lel Qi Gong. His practice is an open system, based on the idea of releasing all internal energy to the universe and absorbing fresh universal energy into the body/mind. One simple practice is to place your hands over your navel, palms toward your belly. Now slowly move your hands apart while imagining releasing of energy to the universe. Then slowly bring your hands back toward each other and your belly while imagining absorbing universal energy into your energy field.

Aerobic Exercise, etc.

Aerobic exercise, sports, weightlifting, walking, running may or may not reduce stress. If performed with tense muscles or a tense mind, energy may be blocked instead of released. Attitude is all-important! If you enjoy it—do it. If not, find another way!

Massage and Polarity Therapy

Massage, Polarity Therapy, and other bodywork and energy work systems help relax the body and mind. Find a practitioner in your area and invest in your health and well-being through regular sessions.

Quick Techniques to Relax the Body

Use your imagination to develop quick relaxation techniques. Take a walk outdoors, jump up and down, get in your car and laugh out loud to exercise and relax your stomach muscles. There is no wrong or right way to relax. The important thing is to give the body a message that says: "It is now time to relax"—and then the reinforcement to do so. Try some of the quick techniques listed below. *Happy relaxing!*

- Give yourself a nightly foot massage. Use an herbal foot balm and gently rub the tender areas. The results will amaze you!
- Take time to massage yourself using a natural oil or lotion. Scent it with the aroma oil that suits your mood—lavender and rose are great stress relievers!
- Massage your mate! My husband and I give each other a five-minute backrub daily to de-stress and feel great!
- Scent your home or work environment with calming and loving fragrances.
- Play relaxing or motivating music in the background. You do not have to listen to "slow" music to relax. There are pieces of classical music designed for inspiration, motivation, and productivity that energize while relaxing! Explore the type of music that relaxes you, and then listen to it often.

Five

Meditation as a Tool for Action

In meditation we hold steady the five senses (seeing, hearing, smelling, tasting, and touching), plus the five powers of action (thinking, talking, handling, walking, and eliminating). This allows the surface mind (which usually takes messages from and sends directions back to the senses and powers) to reverse its orientation.

When the surface mind is no longer distracted by the external world, three things happen:

- The mind calms (as when wind dies down allowing rough water to become calm and sediment to settle again to the bottom).
- Inner features now become objects of attention.
- One reaches ecstasy, or "being outside (*ek*) one's (ordinary) place (*stasis*)."

This results in new perceptions and experiences; new more holistic ways of understanding; a release from ordinary self concerns, anxieties, woes, and habits, allowing other ways of feeling and seeing to develop.

When the five senses become calmed,
Along with the surface mind
And the deep mind wavers not,
That, say the wise, is the deepest state of consciousness.
That state they claim is realized through meditation.
Being the steady-holding of the powers of sense and action.
Then one becomes undistracted:
Indeed, meditation is the beginning and the end!

—*Katha Upanishad 6.10 and 11*
from *Riding the Ox Home*
by Willard Johnson

It is for this purpose that we meditate. To allow ourselves to experience our lives differently, to make new decisions, to grow and develop in peace and love instead of struggle and want.

In the West, meditation has earned a bad reputation. Associated with religion or mysticism, meditation's physical and emotional benefits have often been ignored. The following is a summary of research on meditation; proof that meditation has great value for today's life and well being!

Physiology of Meditation

Studies have shown positive physiological changes during meditation. Here are a few examples.

- Oxygen consumption can be lowered during twenty to thirty minutes of meditation to a degree ordinarily reached only after six to seven hours of sleep (Wallace, Benson, & Wilson [1971] "A wakeful hypometabolic state" *American Journal of Physiology,* 221, 795–799).
- Heart rates and respiration rates typically decrease during meditation [Allison, 1970] "respiratory changes during the practice of transcendental meditation, *Lancet,* 7651, 833–834).
- Forearm blood flow and forehead skin temperatures increase (shift toward parasympathetic dominance). (Ritterstaedt & Schenkluhn, as cited in Kanneliakos [1974] "The Psychobiology of Transcendental Meditation," Menlo Park, CA: W. A. Benjamin).
- Electroencephalograph (EEG) shows an alert-drowsy pattern with high alpha and occasional theta wave patterns, as well as an unusual pattern of swift shifts from alpha to slower (more sleeplike) frequencies and then back again (suggests that meditation may be an unusually fluid state of consciousness, partaking of the qualities of both sleep and wakefulness. (Carrington [1984], p. 112 in Woolfolk and Lehrer, *Principles and Practice of Stress Management*).

Medical Implications of Meditation

Studies have looked at meditation in relation to disease (dis-ease) and found significant benefits to health in healing in meditation. For example:

- Meditation reduces essential hypertension. In one study, twenty patients who had been known to be hypertensive for at least a year, and whose conditions were controlled on antihypertensive medications were treated by relaxation-meditation behavior modification program. In the treatment group, during a three-month trial period, five patients stopped taking their drugs altogether, seven patients showed reductions in drug intake ranging from 33 percent to 66 percent of initial levels, four patients showed better control of blood pressure with medication, and four patients had no difference. Mean systolic blood pressures decreased by 20mm Hg, and mean diastolic blood pressures decreased by 14mm Hg. In a twelve-month follow-up, blood pressure and drug reductions were maintained in those who continued some form of practice of meditation. (Patel [1984] in Woolfolk and Leherer, *Principles and Practice of Stress Management*).
- Meditation significantly reduces airway resistance and demonstrates subjective improvement in bronchial asthma (Wilson, Honaberger, Chiu & Novey [1975]. "Transcendental Meditation and Asthma," *Respiration,* 32, p. 74–80).
- Meditation reduces insomnia (Miskinan, Woolfolk, et al., 1977).
- Meditation reduces stuttering (McIntyre, Silverman, and Trotter, 1974).
- Meditation reduces headaches (Benson, Klenchuk, and Graham 1974).
- Meditation contributes to the reduction in drug abuse, including heroin addiction, alcoholism, and cigarette smoking (Benson, 1969; Benson and Wallace, 1972; Petel and Carruthers, 1977; Shafii, Lavey, and Jaffe, 1974, 1975).

- Meditation is an effective tool in the management of stress (Carrington, Collings, Benson, Robinson, Wood, Lehrer, Woolfolk, and Cole, 1980; Patel, 1975).
- Meditation has resulted in the reduction of premature ventricular contractions in patients with ischemic heart disease (Benson, Alexander, and Feldman, 1975).
- Meditation has reduced serum cholesterol levels in hypercholesterolemic patients (Cooper and Aygen, 1979).
- Meditation has reduced symptoms of psychiatric illness (Glueck and Strooebel, 1975).

Clinical Conditions that Respond to Meditation

(Complete references found in Carrington, 1984 and in Woolfolk and Lehrer, *Principles and Practice of Stress Management,* Guilford Press, New York.)

Reduction in Tension and Anxiety

"While the relaxation brought about by drugs may slow the person down and cause grogginess, the relaxation resulting from meditation does not bring with it any loss of alertness. On the contrary, meditation seems, if anything, to sharpen alertness. Groups of meditators have been shown to have faster reaction times (Appelle and Oswald, 1974) to have better refinement of auditory perception (Pirot, 1978), and to perform more rapidly and accurately on perceptual-motor tasks (Riml, 1978) than nonmeditation controls."

Improvement in Stress-related Illnesses

Meditation is correlated with lessening the severity of many "dis-ease" states, including hypertension and ischemic heart disease (Benson, Alexander, and Feldman, 1975), insomnia (Miskiman, 1978), psychiatric illness (Glueck and Stroebel, 1975) and asthma (Wilson, Honsberger, Chui, and Novey, 1975).

Increased Productivity

Including "lessened need for daytime naps, increased physical stamina, increased productivity on the job, increased ideational fluency, the dissolution of writers' or artists' block, or the release of hitherto unsuspected creative potentials" (Carrington, 1984).

Lessening of Self-Blame

"A spontaneous change in the nature of the meditator's self-statements—from self-castigating to self-accepting—suggests that the noncritical state experienced during the meditation session itself can generalize to daily life" (Carrington, 1984).

Anti-addictive Effects

A series of studies (Benson and Wallace, 1971; Shafii, Lavely, and Jaffee, 1974, 1975) have shown that, at least in persons who continue meditation for long periods of time (usually for a year or more), there may be a marked decease in the use of nonprescription drugs, such as marijuana, amphetamines, barbiturates, and psychedelic substances.

Mood Elevation

People suffering from mild chronic depression or from reactive depression may experience distinct elevation of mood after commencing meditation.

Increase in Available Affect

Release of emotions such as pleasure, sadness, anger, love that have been previously unavailable may occur during meditation sessions or between sessions and . . . may be associated with the recovery of memories that are highly charged emotionally.

Increased Sense of Identity

Meditators have changed from "field-dependent/outer directed to field-independent/inner directed" during meditation practice, thus becoming more aware of their own opinions and being able to arrive at decisions quickly and easily.

Lowered Irritability

The meditating person may become markedly less irritable in his or her interpersonal relationships within a relatively short period of time after commencing meditation.

Limitations of Meditation

Meditation has few limits. It requires no equipment and is possible to do in any environment. Meditation does, however, allow one to "look inside" at the contents of his or her mind. Sometimes these contents are frightening. Negative memories, judgments, and guilt may rise to the surface. The point of meditation is to release this mental content, so by following the practice of nonattachment these negatives can be quickly released. Meditation is not psychoanalysis. It is important to not become caught up in the content. It's the pure process of discovering the True Self that is the goal. With this said, the following are some limitations of meditation.

Tension-Release Side Effects

- . . . physiological and/or psychological symptoms of a temporary nature may appear during or following meditation . . . caused by the release of deep-seated nonverbal tension.

In meditation we access deeper levels of our consciousness and some of these levels contain painful memories. By learning how to observe these memories and then let them go in the present moment, we are able to perform a clearing and cleansing both mentally and physically. This process may cause some discomfort, but passes quickly as we gain new control over our thoughts and feelings.

Rapid Behavior Change

- Meditation may foster a form of self-assertion that conflicts with an already established neurotic solution of being overly self-effacing.

This is a true story about the effects of meditation on one family. A hard working wife and mother visited her doctor because of high blood pressure. The doctor had just been reading research on meditation and knew of a local program for his patient. The woman enrolled and learned to perform a simple, daily practice of meditation. One month later, she returned to her doctor with her blood pressure nicely under control. However, her family asked to speak with the doctor in private. "What did you do to her?" They asked. "She used to be so agreeable to every request we had. She was great at picking up our clothes and cooking extra meals and waiting on us. Now, she wants us to do some of the work. She wants equal rights in this house and we don't like it!" By experiencing the peace and comfort of meditation, this wife and mother learned to re-claim her individual place in the home. Instead of being a martyr and "stuffing her feelings into high blood pressure" she learned to say "no." She learned that she was worthy in her own right, and did not need to please others all the time to feel valuable. This is a true shift and change in her lifestyle, leading to a longer and healthier life.

- Meditation tends to bring about feelings of well-being and optimism, which may threaten the playing out of a depressive role.

If you enjoy being depressed, then do not meditate! Meditation leads us into our center of joy and optimism. Meditation brings the world into balance and harmony. Meditation changes our outlook and perspective and moves us toward the positive and happy.

- The deeply pleasurable feelings that can accompany or follow a meditation session can cause anxiety.

Many of us have learned to worry about feeling too good. We repeat lines such as, "This is too good to be true—wait until the other shoe drops." Feeling good can cause us to become anxious about the bad that is sure to come. These notions are pure nonsense. Feeling good is a foreign experience to some people. If it is for you, remind yourself that you want to experience this new state often, that you are learning how to feel differently, and that these new, pleasurable feelings will become natural with time and practice.

Meditation can result in an easing of life pace, which may threaten to alter a fast-paced, high-pressured life style that is used neurotically as a defense or in the service of drives for power, achievement, or control.

In other words, meditation may result in changes in lifestyle and the experience of new ways of being in the world. For some, this change brings anxiety. For people ready to change and grow, meditation is a life-affirming experience.

Cautions

Some people may be hypersensitive to meditation and must begin with small five-to-ten minute daily sessions, or meditate initially only once a week until tolerance is developed.

Release of emotional material that is difficult to handle may occur with prolonged meditation (three to four hours).

Meditation may enhance the action of certain drugs, reducing the requirements for antianxiety and antidepressive drugs as well as antihypertensive and thyroid-regulating medications. Therefore, if you are taking medication, consult with your prescribing physician if you find you need to decrease the dosage of current drugs.

Other chapters explore foundational theories and practices of the three major forms of meditation. For now, here are five ways you can begin your meditation practice. Select one, and stick with it. Perform it daily for five minutes and experience the results for yourself.

Breathing: Breathe in to a mental count of four, hold for four, breath out for four, hold for four (this is a technique you can do anywhere, anytime, to relax).

Mindfulness: Feel your breath as it comes in through your nose and goes out through your nose. Stay with the breath. Note each thought you have and imagine it in a bubble of air, floating to the surface and breaking free. Observe the thought bubble and let it go. Practice this ten minutes each day.

Music: Listen to music that relaxes you—*really listen,* sitting in a comfortable position, with your eyes closed. Do not *do* anything while listening; just *be* with the music.

Visualize the positive and the relaxing: During a quiet time, close your eyes and imagine you are sitting in a place in nature that is very relaxing for you. It may be a place you have been before, or one you only can imagine being at. Let yourself sense, feel, taste, smell, see, and hear that place. Let your body relax, let your mind relax; let yourself spend some time at peace.

Affirmations: Use the information from the chapter 3 to create an affirmation. Repeat one over and over as you are going to bed. Try to let a positive affirmation be the last thing you think about at night. Then, in the morning, repeat it over and over as you are getting ready for your day. The classic affirmation is:

"Every day, in every way, my life is getting better and better!"

Six

Meditation Techniques Overview

Now that you know why meditation is good for you, let us discover how to meditate. The best definition I have for meditation is that it is **a skill or technique involving the development of inward aspects of consciousness in order to enhance one's abilities to attain one's life goals.** That's right—it is a technique to do better in the world!

Without the ability to maintain an inner calm, our ventures in the world become chaotic. In meditation, we go inward to find the Source of Life, we bathe in that Source, we renew in that Source, and then we return to the world to "do good." A daily practice of meditation enables us to bring love, peace, joy, and all the other positive attributes into our lives and the lives of those around us. We give to others what we have inside. In meditation, we learn that inside is peace and love. And that is what we then can give to our families, our work, our community, and our world. Powerful stuff!

For clarity, I have divided all meditation techniques into one of three categories or types of meditation: concentration, contemplation, and mindfulness. These are arbitrary divisions, useful in exploring each general type in depth. At the end of this chapter is a chart outlining the types presented below.

Concentration Meditation

Concentration meditation includes forms of meditation that require concentration on a single object or concept. In this form, we focus our undivided attention on some "thing" to the exclusion of all other "things" in our world.

Elements

- Requires the highest mental concentration and involves the calming of all mental processes.

Process

- We maintain an increasing concentrated focus of attention on a single object.

Results

- Temporary attainment of altered states of consciousness (alpha, theta and delta brain waves).

Brain Wave Frequencies—A Brief Explanation

We all go into "altered states of consciousness" daily. Our normal brain wave patterns range from beta when we are active and thinking and reacting to the world around us, to alpha when we begin to relax, back up to beta when we are stimulated, and down to alpha again when we begin to go to sleep at night. During sleep, we alternate between alpha and theta, with occasional trips to delta.

In meditation, we learn to control or direct these frequencies to a certain extent. Instead of them "just happening to us," we choose to go to alpha, and we do so. The issue is not whether we go into these states, it is that we journey there when we desire to!

Brain Wave Frequencies

Beta = 14–21 cps = objective, material world of effect.

Alpha = 7–14 cps = subjective, spiritual world of cause.

Theta = 4–7 cps = controls autonomic nervous system and normalizes cells, tissues, organs, and glands.

Delta = < 4 cps = deep, dreamless state of being.

Examples of Concentration Meditation Techniques

- Concentrate on an *IMAGE.* Focus on a candle, a painting, a sunset, a tree, a crystal. The focus is exclusively on the image. Just sit and focus. When thoughts distract the mind, return to the focus. Continually returning to the focus until you are there!

- Concentrate on a *SOUND.* Focus your attention on the sound of waves breaking on the sand, of a babbling brook, of the pure chant of the universal sound of OM. If you are not into "OM-ing" it, try this exercise. Sit by yourself or invite a friend to join you. Now sing the vowels! Sing "Aaaaaaaaa" three times, putting your soul into the sound. (The tone doesn't matter at this point, just sing!) Now sing, "Eeeeeeee" three times, then "Iiiiiiiiii, Ooooooo," and finally, "Uuuuuuuu." Notice how you felt before you began to sing, and how you feel after. Pick your favorite vowel sound and sing it for five minutes, then for ten minutes. You are meditating!

Where Is There?

Our normal consciousness, what we call "thinking" involves an awareness of dualism. Something is "that," but not "this." In meditation, we are able to go beyond this dualism into pure awareness. Philosophers call this space the void, the "no-thing." Nondualistic awareness attained during meditation is a space of no conflicts, because there are no opposites. This special space of Being fills us with peace.

Meditation Continuum:
Thinking . . . Visualizing . . .
Experiencing . . . Being
Dualistic awareness of . . .
nondualistic pure awareness

- Concentrate on an *IDEA.* Repeat the word "love," "peace," "joy," or "health," over and over. Say it out loud. Say it silently. Repeat it until you go past its concept and discover its feeling and meaning.

- Concentrate on a *PRECEPT.* The traditional form of concentration meditation is the *mantra.* A mantra is a vehicle for transporting the mind beyond thought. Chapter 9 explores the art of mantra meditation.

- Concentrate on a *SENSATION.* If sitting outdoors, focus on the feeling of the wind on your cheek. Or focus on your breath as it comes in and out through your nose. We will explore this technique more in chapters 7 and 8 on mindfulness meditation.

Contemplation Meditation

Contemplation Meditation includes forms of meditation that require concentration on a variety of concepts, selecting some and excluding others. This is broader than that of concentration meditation, yet there is an inward focus to the exclusion of outward stimuli.

Elements

- Development of access concentration through a selected concentration meditation technique.
- The creation of thoughts or images within the mind.

Process

- Attention is focused upon an image or feeling/thought to the exclusion of all other stimuli.

Results

- Change experienced in the outer, objective world as a result of these inner, subjective experiences.

Examples of Contemplation Meditation Techniques

Affirmations

Affirmations are developed and repeated over and over (see chapter 3 in this section for the development of personal affirmations).

Visualization and Guided Imagery

Often called "self-hypnosis," imagery is used to effect change in the outer world. Athletes use imagery to mentally rehearse performance for greater results. Healing imagery can stimulate the body's response to stress, pain and "dis-ease." A wonderful book for dealing with health problems is Gerald Epstein's *Healing*

Visualizations: Creating Health Through Imagery. In this book Dr. Epstein lists hundreds of three-to five minute visualizations he has used to help his patients heal from the common cold to more serious diseases. We will explore specific techniques for visualization in chapter 10.

Prayer

This is the oldest form of contemplation meditation. Simple, sincere prayer to your Source works wonders. Prayer is a potent form of meditation and can be practiced anytime, anywhere.

Koan Meditation

Koan meditation originates in Japan. A Koan is a riddle that must be contemplated upon until the answer reveals itself. A common Koan is, "What is the sound of one hand clapping?" The answer comes not from our dualistic mind, but from our deeper mind. Years may be spent in Koan contemplation. My favorite Koan is "What did you look like before your parents were born?" Trying to answer this question sends the mind spinning back and back until, exhausted, it gives up and access to the Higher Self is provided.

Inquiry

This is another form of potent contemplation meditation. In inquiry, you sit, relax, and then begin to ask yourself, "Who am I?" Accept any answers that come, but do not dwell on them. Then repeat the question, "Who am I?" Again, wait for the answers to come, and then repeat the question. Eventually, if you stick with it, you will enter an area of truth and wisdom deep within yourself.

Mindfulness Meditation

Mindfulness meditation includes forms of meditation that require nonattached awareness of all thoughts, sensations, and feelings. Nothing is excluded from your awareness. The emphasis is on the observation, without judgment of all phenomena.

Elements

- Development of access concentration through a selected concentration meditation technique.
- Observation of sensory and mental processes without attachment.

Process

- Complete, direct, and immediate awareness of all phenomena that presents itself.

Results

- Enduring change through the realization of subject/object dualism and the impermanence of all phenomena.

Explanation of the above sentence: If the Results point above sounded like a Koan to you, that's okay! In mindfulness meditation, you experience (not think about, not analyze, not intellectualize), but experience that all thoughts are dualistic and all thoughts are subject to change. There is an opposite for every thought I have, every word I speak. That's dualism. Every thought I have comes and goes. That's impermanence. When I know this truth in my heart, I can let go of stress, tension, worry, and fear. I learn to know through the experience of mindfulness meditation.

Examples of Contemplation Meditation Techniques

- Become aware of your ***breath*** as it comes and goes through your nose. You may choose to simply count each breath, not trying to influence it, but simply observing and counting. (Note: the chapters 7 and 8 explore this technique in depth!)
- Become aware of your ***thoughts***. Quietly observe each thought that passes through your mind and label it as "past" or "future." It will be one or the

other, because if you are truly centered in the present moment, you will have no thoughts to label!

- Become aware of *sensations* by observing them within the experience of meditation.
- Become aware of *feelings* by going beyond the feeling to experience the space and energy within.

Summary

You have just read a brief overview of meditation techniques. Following chapters will offer in-depth instruction in the practice of Mindfulness Meditation (chapters 7 and 8), Mantra Meditation (chapter 9), Visualization and Guided Imagery (chapter 10). Until then, pick a technique noted above and try it! Spend ten minutes or more each day and see what happens.

Types	Concentration	Contemplation	Mindfulness
Elements	Highest mental concentration Calming of all mental processes	Access concentration Creating thoughts and images	Access concentration Observation of sensory and mental processes
Process	Increasing concentration of focus and attention on a single object	Attention focused upon an image or feeling or thought to the exclusion of other stimuli	Complete, direct, and immediate awareness of all phenomena that presents itself
Results	Temporary attainment of altered states of consciousness (alpha, theta, and delta brain wave states)	Change experienced in the outer, objective world as a result of the inner, subjective experience.	Enduring change by realization of subject/object dualism and the impermanence of phenomena
Examples	Concentration on a . . . . . . Precept (Mantra) . . . Image (Candle, crystal, painting, nature) . . . Sound (Waves, OM) . . . Idea (Love, peace) . . . Sensation (Breath)	Mind directed to a particular arena . . . . . . Visualization and Guided Imagery (Peaceful beach) . . . Affirmations ("I love and accept myself now") . . . Prayer ("Not my will but Thy will be done") . . . Koan ("What did you look like before your parents were born?") . . . Inquiry ("Who am I?")	Awareness of inward phenomena including . . . . . . Breath (Breath counting) . . . Thoughts (Thought labeling) . . . Sensations (Observing the thought/feeling within the sensation) . . . Feelings (Going through feelings to sense neutral energy within)

Table 3. Meditation Techniques

Seven

The Practice of Mindfulness

Stop a moment before reading on. What is on your mind *right now?* Are you wondering what this chapter is all about? Are you thinking about what you are going to do next? Or are you thinking about what you just did?

Our minds contain thousands and thousands of thoughts each day. Each thought has a direct impact on our emotions and on our bodies. Rarely do we experience the present moment. We are locked in the past or planning the future. When was the last time you were truly mindful of the moment? The usual answer is, "When I was on vacation and I saw a beautiful sunset. I was just there!"

It is Possible to Be on Vacation Every Day

The skill involved is the practice of mindfulness. In mindfulness, we observe inward, watching our thoughts without attachment to them, similar to lying on the grass and watching the clouds go by. This art of nonattachment to our thoughts results in great healing, peace, and insight. Author and researcher Jon Kabat-Zinn *(Full Catastrophe Living, Wherever You Go, There You Are)* has demonstrated through research that simply by being mindful of physical and mental pain we can overcome, or rather come through, and experience peace.

The Practice is Quite Simple

To begin, set your timer or stopwatch for five minutes. Then sit in a comfortable position, close your eyes, and focus on your breath. *Feel* the breath coming and going, going and coming, through your nose. Your breath becomes the vehicle to carry you toward peace. Now notice how easily you become distracted from the feel of your breath. A thought travels through your mind. That thought leads to another, and another.

Finally, you remember that you are supposed to be feeling your breath, and you return. But from where did you return? Where does the mind go? Experiment again and this time you feel a pressure or pain in your body. You follow that pain and another series of thoughts results, and again, you return to the breath. Each time you return to the sensation of your own breath on your nose you have gained a little more control over your own mind.

Our Own Mind Carries Us Away

Our thoughts are like unruly children, constantly pulling us here and there. This constant pulling is the source of our stress and pain. Mindfulness is the skill that allows us to watch our thoughts and feelings without being pulled by them. Initially in practice all this mental chatter preoccupies us. Then we begin to realize that we do have control. By noticing and observing, we stop reacting. It is our reactions to our thoughts that bring us emotional stress and physical dis-ease.

Mindfulness requires of us, and develops in us, the following qualities:

- *Nonjudging*—becoming an impartial witness to your own experience.
- *Patience.*
- *Beginner's mind*—a willingness to see everything as if for the first time.
- *Trust in yourself.*
- *Nonstriving*—by doing nothing all is done.
- *Acceptance*—seeing things as they actually are in the present.
- *Letting go.*

When you are ready, lengthen your five-minute practice to ten minutes, twenty minutes, or more. Experiencing longer practice periods will allow you to enter a space beyond your thoughts. This is the space of energy before it is bound up within a thought. Deepak Chopra, M.D. *(Ageless Body, Timeless Mind, Unconditional Life, Wisdom Within),* describes this inner space as a "void of pure possibilities, impulses of energy and information," and "a space made up of nothing, the womb of creation." Direct experience of this "void of no-thing" can have a transformative and profoundly healing effect on body, emotion, mind, and life. So are you ready? Set aside at least five minutes *every* day to sit and feel your breath. Enjoy your practice!

Eight

Deepening the Practice of Mindfulness

Meditation, as written about in the Katha Upanishad (400–300 B.C.), describes the essential Self as a chariot owner, the body as the chariot, the deep mind as the charioteer, and the surface mind as the reins. Our powers of sensation and action are the horses and the objects we interact with are the fields upon which the chariot travels. The only way to control the whole mechanism is through meditation. In meditation, the Self is contacted. This higher Self guides the mind and body that in turn guides the chariot to where we wish to go in life. Without the mental awareness and control developed through meditation, we are constantly out of control. A more modern analogy is that of

Katha Upanishad

The essential Self is the chariot owner, understand,
The body only the chariot;
The deep mind see as the charioteer,
And the surface mind as the reins.

The powers of sense and action are the horses, they say,
And the sense objects the fields where they travel.
Those who know say; the body, powers of sense and action,
And the surface mind are the experience mechanism.

Indeed, who is not mentally aware,
Whose surface mind is forever undisciplined,
That person's powers of sense and action will be out of control,
Like mean horses uncontrolled by a charioteer.

But whoever becomes aware,
With surface mind always disciplined by meditation,
That person's powers of sense and action will be under control,
Like good horses, under the charioteer's control.

getting into a taxicab and telling the driver that we want to go north. A second later we tell the driver we wish to go south. A second after that we decide to go west, then east. Steady control is required to guide our experience mechanisms, be they taxi cabs or chariots, through life.

Most of us spend most of our days out of control! We have so many thoughts that send us into the past or into the future and take away our present moment of power. Mindfulness meditation allows us to contact the present, and empowers us to creative action.

How Can I Control My Thoughts?

Most of the time we identify with the surface mind, the reins. We think that our thoughts are who we are. Yet there is a deeper self who is holding the reins, and there is an even deeper self who owns the chariot. Or, if you like a more modern analogy, we identify with the taxicab, the steering wheel, and the road, forgetting that we are paying for the ride and can direct the cab where we please. In the practice of mindfulness we observe our thoughts, sensations, and feelings without becoming attached to them. We assert control by letting go of all the surface clutter and by realizing that all these things going on are not us.

What Am I Doing with All These Thoughts?

Steven Levine, in his book *A Gradual Awakening,* uses the metaphor of a train to describe thoughts and thinking. Imagine standing on the roadside, watching a train go by. Each boxcar on the train contains a thought. In one boxcar there is the thought about the rent due next week. In another is a thought about what you are going to have for dinner tonight. The goal of the practice of mindfulness is to see the landscape beyond the train. We begin to meditate. We focus on our breath, coming and going. We feel the breath at the nostrils. We begin to see the landscape. Then suddenly a boxcar thought goes by. In this boxcar we are arguing with our boss. We hop aboard that boxcar and we are off and down the track. One thought leads to another, and to another. We are far and away from following our breath, from seeing the landscape.

So What Do I Do in Practice?

Begin by finding a comfortable place where you will not be disturbed. One student of mine put a big pillow in the bathroom and meditated there. It was the only place in the house where she had any privacy! Set a timer for twenty minutes or more, then set it away from you so you will not be tempted to "peek" to see how much time is left. Close your eyes and focus on your breath. Feel the breath coming and going, going and coming from your nose. Simply observe your breathing. Do not try to control it. When you find yourself distracted from the breath, you may try the following.

Distracted by Thoughts and Feelings

Try labeling each thought and feeling. Use such labels as "future thought," "past thought," "angry feeling," "loving feeling." As soon as you have labeled the thought, return immediately to the sensation of your breath.

Distracted by Sensations

Avoid the tendency to respond to sensations. Do not scratch an itch or adjust position because of a discomfort. Notice the itch as "itch" and the discomfort as "pain." And return immediately to the sensation of your breath. The mind cannot calm down if the body is in constant motion. If you are really in an awkward position, then mindfully change that position and return to your breath.

How Will All This Benefit Me?

Over a period of time, with consistent daily practice, you will naturally become less responsive to and more responsible for the contents of your mind. Consistent practice is essential. You cannot learn how to play tennis if you only go to the courts once a month for twenty minutes. Meditation is a skill and a habit. Once you have developed both, you will not want to be without them. There are some added benefits. Try extending your practice time to forty minutes, or even one hour, once a week. You may find yourself traveling to the landscape completely beyond thought—a wonderful place of pure healing, light, and love. But don't expect it! An expectation is just a thought, and thoughts keep us from experiencing the light of pure awareness. The bottom line is that we are more than our thoughts. Thoughts are just encapsulated energy. The experience of Essential Self, our state of pure energy, will heal and free us to grow and serve.

Nine

Concentration Meditation

Forms of concentration meditation have been practiced in India, Tibet, and the East for ages. Concentration meditation was popularized in the West in the form of mantras used by Maharishi Mahesh Yogi in the 1960s, and trademarked as TM (Transcendental Meditation™).

Attention by the medical community came in the 1970s through Herbert Benson, M.D. Dr. Benson studied the techniques of TM and "Westernized" them into a formula of practice for inducing the "relaxation response" (see Benson's *The Relaxation Response* and *Beyond the Relaxation Response*).

Most Western medical research findings are based on subjects using one of the various forms of concentration or mantra meditation.

Traditional Posture

The traditional posture for meditation is called the "Seven Gestures":

- Sitting with legs crossed, pelvis elevated on a pillow (or sitting in a chair with feet flat on the floor).
- Hands resting on knees (palms up or palms down).
- Spine balanced without being rigid.

- Chin slightly tucked in.
- Eyes gazing downward (or closed or gazing slightly up).
- Mouth slightly open with jaw relaxed.
- Tip of tongue touching palate ridge just behind upper teeth.

By following these postures, a stillness is induced within the body, making the quieting of the mind easier.

Concentration on a Sound

A mantra, or specific sound, is used as a "vehicle for the mind" to ride upon to attain deeper states of concentration and being. In Transcendental Meditation (TM), the sound mantra is selected by the instructor to vibrate with the student in a special way. Mantras usually have no meaning to the meditator, but the sound quality is conductive to producing deep rest and refined awareness. Try the following sounds, out loud, and experiment with the note and rhythm of them to find the best tones for your healing and well being.

Examples of sounds:

- OM (AUM, AMEN, AMIN, HUM)—universal sound of awareness (AH OU-MM: using three-part breath).
- HU—sound of love, balance, and harmony.
- AH—sound of emotion, desire, and creativity.
- EH (EE)—sound of soul force and universal life.

When the sound is "sung" out loud, the combined effect of the deep breathing required to produce the sound, with the tonal qualities of the sound itself produces profound relaxation. The sound may also be repeated silently, in harmony with the breath.

Concentration on a Word or Phrase

The following general procedure may be followed during this form of meditation.

- Select a word of phrase that reflects your belief system (a line from a prayer, a concept such as love, peace, joy; an affirmation; an image of peace).
- Choose a comfortable position.
- Close your eyes.
- Relax your muscles from feet to head.
- Be aware of your breathing, and begin to repeat the word or phrase (silently or out loud).
- Maintain a passive attitude.
- Continue for a set period of time (ten-to-twenty minutes).
- Practice the technique twice a day.

Traditional Phrases

- Gate, Gate, Paragate, Parasumgate, Bodhi, Suaha (GAH-TAY, GAH-TAY, PAH-R-GAH-TAY, PAH-R-SRUM GAH-TAY BOW-DEE SWAH-HAH)—Buddhist for "Beyond, Beyond, the Great Beyond, Beyond that Beyond, to Thee Homage.
- OM Namaha Shivaya—(OM, NA-MAH, SHE-VI-A) Sanskrit for " I honor the God/Goddess within."
- Aum Mani Padme Hum—(AH-OWM MAH-NAY PAUD-MAY HOOM)—Tibetan for "The All is a precious jewel in the lotus flower which blooms in my heart."
- "Hail Mary, full of grace . . ."—Christian/Catholic.

- "Our Father, who art in Heaven . . ."—or any line from the Lord's Prayer.
- "Not my will, but Thine be done . . ."—or any meaningful spiritual phrase.

Modern Mantras

Construct your own mantra by creating a six-to-ten syllable phrase that is personally meaningful and repeated effortlessly in rhythm to the breath.

Examples include:

- "The waves roll in and roll out."
- "Returning to my center."
- "River flowing into the sea."
- "Peace is with me now."
- "I'm willing to change and grow."
- "I relax, I release, I let go."

Concentration on an Object

Gently watch, in a unfocused manner, the light from a candle, a scene in nature, the clouds, a symbol, a statue, or a drawing.

Concentration on a Sensation

Experience the inflowing and outflowing of the breath by concentrating on the sensation of breathing either at the abdomen (rising and falling) or at the nostrils (air moving in and out).

Summary

Mantras can be as complex and sacred, or as simple and joyous as you wish. The first mantra I heard was long ago on the Moody Blues album *In Search of the Lost Chord*. On one song, they sang, "Aaaa Aaaa Ummmm," over and over. I was entranced. This was long before I had ever heard of meditation. Several years ago my husband and I studied with an Indian Swami (a type of guru or holy man) who gave us a personal mantra. Another time, a Sufi holy man instructed me in a healing mantra. I use all at different times (what would the Moody Blues say!).

The most important point is to find a sound or phrase that "feels good" to you. When you say it out loud or silently, allow a feeling of peace and surrender and protection come to you, and then use it! If you wish help getting started, I recommend the following CDs:

- *Chakra Chants* by Jonathan Goldman is *the best* music we've ever experienced for aligning and balancing the chakras. The CD has seven tracks, one for each chakra. They are recorded using the keynote, frequency, vowel, Bija, element, Shabd sound, instrument and energy for each chakra. Listening to this CD daily has a profound effect on body, mind, and spirit. We know we are changing and growing through its use.
- *The Crimson Collection* interweaves celestial vocals by Singh Kaur with Kim Robertson's stunning instrumental textures on Celtic harp and keyboards. The eighty minutes of repeated Sikh mantras have the power to induce a deep state of serenity in the listener.
- Robert Gass and *On Wings of Song* have recorded many chanting tapes. *Songs of Healing* is our favorite! Stephen Levine has written about "healing unto life or death," and this album captures that theme. These songs

allow healing to occur, even acknowledging dying as the ultimate healing (listen to the first song, whose words are: *"Go in Beauty, Peace be with you until we meet again in the Light."*

Practice "singing" the sound or phrase out loud—alone or with others. Repeat it silently while meditating or just before going to sleep at night. Find the time to go within and you will be truly amazed at the results!

OM

Ten

Guided Imagery and Visualization

Visualization is the process we use to form a mental "picture" of the world. This "seeing with the mind's eye" may involve actual seeing, or imaging, or pretending, or feeling, or knowing, or sensing—the mode differs with each person.

To discover your mode of visualizing, close your eyes after reading this sentence and visualize a pink elephant . . . what direction was he/she facing? However you were able to determine the direction of the elephant is your current mode of visualizing. Some people clearly "see" the elephant in their minds. Others simple "know" in which direction the elephant was facing. It's like reading a book. How do you picture the characters? Would you recognize them on the street? There is no wrong or right way to visualize. Just do it and accept your mode as correct for you.

Think about the past, and you're visualizing.
Imagine the future—you're visualizing too!
Read a book, listen to music, and even think a thought!
All part of the visualizing you!

Guided Imagery

Guided imagery is a technique used by oneself or another to direct visualization in specific ways by describing a scene that you imagine (visualize) as clearly as you can. Examples of scenes are: a mountain setting, images of yourself as a successful person, or pictures of what an emotion might look like.

Guided imagery may be used to:

Foster empathy	*Set goals*	*Enhance creativity*
Manage stress	*Rehearse the future*	*Practice a skill*
Improve performance	*Relieve pain, fear*	*Control habits*
Promote personal growth	*Enhance learning*	*Promote healing*

Recent purposes of guided imagery and visualization include:

- Discover or change subconscious "programs."
- Mentally practice motor skills and performances.
- Relax and transform reactions into responses.
- Connect with others.
- Connect with one's Higher (Inner or Deeper) Self.

Let me take you on a trip.
We'll not use cars or boats or planes.
Come journey with me through the imagination of your mind.
To places wonderful to discover and joyous to find!

Steps in Using Guided Imagery to Create a Special Place

- Go through a relaxation exercise or appropriate imagery.
- Mentally create a "safe place" in nature that you will return to each time you use the visualization.
- Include a dwelling to decorate, and a screen or window on which to view your images.
- Use a combination of PROJECTIVE techniques (you are consciously creating the scenes before you) and RECEPTIVE techniques (you are open to receive images from the subconscious and supraconscious mind).
- Conclude with an energizing exercise or imagery.

The following is a guided imagery that you may practice. Read the imagery into a tape recorder and listen to it or have a friend read it to you. This imagery contains all the steps to using imagery for healing and "Well Being."

Basic Guided Imagery

Begin by taking a deep breath, in through the bottoms of your feet, out through the top of your head and your fingertips. Now take a second breath, in through your feet and out through your head. Then, take a third breath.

Imagine, pretend, or feel that there is a ball of light about six inches above the top of your head. It is a ball of warm light. You can see it as a white light or you may even see it as a different color. It is about six inches above the top of your head and, in a moment, you will be bringing that light into your head to relax your body. Feel the light now coming into the top of your head and entering into your forehead. Your forehead and scalp relax as the light touches them. The back of your head relaxes, almost as if, where the light touches, an internal massage, and internal balancing is occurring. The light caresses the cells and tissues in your face and you watch yourself relax with the light.

You feel the light now flowing down into your eyes and eyelids. Your eyeballs feel as if they are relaxing, being massaged. The temples and back of your head are relaxing. Light goes down now into your cheeks, and your jaws relax. Your ears are warm and relaxed. The back of your head is warm and relaxed. Feel the relaxation occurring, feel the balancing occurring. The light now flows down your throat and the back of your neck. Your throat relaxes. You may wish to swallow. Swallowing will only take you deeper into relaxation.

Allow the light now to flow across the tops of your shoulders, giving an internal massage to the muscles that are on the tops of your shoulders, feeling and relaxing even more. Feel the warmth of circulation, growing relaxation. The light flows now down your arms to your elbows, forearms, wrist, hands, and fingers. As this warmth, this light, this relaxation flows, you may even feel a slight tingling in your fingertips. Allow your arms to relax, allow the cells and tissues to relax.

The light now flows to the base of your throat, then it begins to expand through your chest and upper back. Each place the light touches becomes more balanced, more whole, more healed. The light expands throughout your chest and breasts, heart and lungs. Allow the light to flow now into your lower back and surround your kidneys, flowing down into your stomach, intestines, and pelvic area. Each place the light touches becomes more balanced and more healed. Light now flowing into your pelvic area, massaging and relaxing, back and front. Cells, tissues, and organs functioning perfectly now. Relax.

The light flows further down the thighs and knees. Deeper and deeper into relaxation. Flowing down into the ankles and feet. Wonderfully relaxed. Now take a moment and send this light to any place in your body that still feels a bit tense. Use your mind, your imagination to send the light to any place of tension, simply by shining the light and notice the release from the tension. Allow the light to flow out through the pores of your skin, surrounding you in a halo, a cocoon of light. A peaceful cocoon of light, just the right temperature. Feeling the light.

Now notice that from this cocoon of light a small bubble of light emerges. Place a portion of your consciousness into this bubble and feel it begin to float up. This bubble is going to be your vehicle for travel into your own mind. As part of you floats up in this bubble of light, you may even be able to look down upon yourself and see yourself from above. A pretty unusual view!

Now let this bubble of light rise up and begin to travel, taking you and your mind to a place that represents peace and beauty and safety for you. Feel yourself traveling now. Across the land. Maybe heading toward the beach, or the mountains, or the river, or the desert. Letting yourself travel toward this place of safety, this place of peace, this place of joy. Seeing it now more clearly in your mind, arriving at this place and stepping out of the bubble.

Look around. What do you see? Look at the sky, what color is it? Are there clouds? What kind of day is it? Are there trees around? What kind of trees? Notice the colors and the textures. What does this place smell like? Is it the saltiness of the ocean, or the deep, earthy scent of the mountains and forest, or the clear, dry scent of the desert? Is there a breeze blowing? What does it feel like on your skin? Reach down and feel what you are standing on. Run the sand through your fingers, or the leaves, or the grass. Another deep breath and just enjoy being here for a moment. Just enjoy letting yourself experience the feelings of this place.

When you are ready, turn around and look behind you. You will see a structure of some sort. It could be a cabin, or a tree house, or a cave or . . . Notice the structure. What is it made of? Are there windows in it? Go now with your mind to the front door. Notice what the door is like. Open the door and walk inside. This is your retreat center, where your most powerful visualizations will occur.

The first thing you want to do is to decorate the inside in the style that is comfortable to you. Stand in the center of the room now and face the north wall. Facing the north wall of the room, notice what is on it. Is it bare wood or painted? What color is it? Are there windows on the north wall, or a fireplace, or a computer system? Are there chairs on the north side of the room? Is there carpeting on the floor, or is it wood or some other material? Decorate the north wall any way you wish. You may place a picture on it if you want to, a certain piece of furniture. It is your wall and you may decorate it any way you want.

When you are ready, turn to the right and face the east wall. Again, notice what is on it and what is near it. Are there windows? Curtains on the windows? Is there a little eating area on the east side? Arrange the east just right for you. When you are ready, turn again and face the south. What is on the south wall? Notice the colors, the textures, and the objects in the south of your room. Again, decorate this area and when you are ready, turn again the face the west wall. Put anything you want to on this wall. Allow images to come, and if they do not, make up your own! Now turn to the center of the room.

In the center of the room is the most comfortable chair you can imagine. It is a chair that you can sit in and feel safe and protected. Notice the color, the texture of your chair. It is a wonderfully cozy chair. Now go and sit down in the chair and snuggle in. Let the chair hold and support your body. Feel how wonderful it feels to be relaxing in this special chair.

Notice now that by your fingertips are two buttons, up and down. Press the down button and a screen comes down in front of you. It's a movie screen, about five or ten feet in front of you—a big, wide, movie screen. This is the screen upon which you are going to do your visualizations.

First we are gong to initiate the screen to make it even more real in our minds. As the screen comes down, you notice that next to you in the chair on the floor is a big bucket of red paint and a big housepainter's brush. Take the brush of red paint and paint your name on the screen, letter by letter. Paint your name on the screen. See the letters clearly stand out on your own screen. When you finish, sit back in your seat. Now we will do a color test pattern on the screen. Mentally change your name that is in red on the screen to orange. See your name changing to orange on the screen. Now change the orange to yellow. And now you see your name in yellow changing to green. The green now changes to blue. Then the blue changes to violet. The violet changes to white now. If your screen is white, and your name is now white, you will see your name fading into the screen. If the screen is black, change your name once more to black and see it fading into the screen.

Now, on the screen, project this morning. See yourself on the screen waking up this morning. Watch yourself waking up. What did you do first? Go through the entire morning from the time you woke up until you arrived at this place of meditation. See it as vividly as possible without strain or tension. You are developing the ability to visualize!

Now place another image on the screen. This time see yourself standing in a meadow, with the forest just beyond it. See yourself standing in that meadow, with the grass blowing in the wind. The sun is out, but not too warm, the temperature is just right. There is a path that winds toward the forest.

At this time, your choice is to sit in your chair and watch yourself walk the path, or, if you wish, get out of your chair and step into the screen so that you now see the path from the perspective of you walking on it—from your own eyes. Begin to walk the path, noticing the wild flowers, feeling the gentle wind. You are now at the edge of the woods. Something shiny and smooth attracts your attention on the path and you reach down to pick it up. You hold it in your hand and look at it. This object is a symbol for you and the symbol tells you something about how to develop your relaxation and meditation ability. It may not be clear to you at this very moment what the symbol means, but thinking about the symbol during the coming week will assist you in learning to relax and meditate at deeper and deeper levels.

Now step back out of the screen and sit down again in the chair and let the image of the meadow fade on the screen. Let one more image go onto the screen, an image of you interacting with someone in the future. See yourself and the other person having an interaction that will come out in a wonderful way for both of you. Feel the happiness between you. It may be that a problem is resolved so both of you are satisfied. It may be that something has been said that needed to be said. Rehearse the scene. You can either be in the scene or watch the scene from your chair. When the scene is over, once again sit down in your chair. Let the image fade from the screen. Press the up button by your fingertips and see the screen returning to the ceiling.

Now stand up from your chair, look around the room, and know that you can come back here anytime you wish, know that each time you come back the room will become more real for you. You will be able to do more decorating. It will represent to your mind the place where imagination, creativity, and work for the highest good of all concerned. Look once more around the room, and then head toward the door, feeling very good about the room you have created. Step out into the scene of nature and feel again the peace that you have when you are here. You deserve to experience this more and more in your life.

Find the bubble that brought you here and step inside. You feel yourself beginning to return to the present. The bubble comes slowly into the room you occupy in the present. You now feel the bubble separating at the bottom of your feet into many smaller bubbles. These bubbles of light are energizing, vitalizing bubbles of light. When they enter the bottoms of your feet, your feet begin to tingle slightly with this energy, this awakening, this aliveness. As the light moves through your feet and ankles, you begin to move your toes and ankles around, feeling more and more energized as the bubble of light moves up into your calves and knees and thighs. Letting the energy come back in, feeling the aliveness of the energy. The energy moving now up into your midsection, up to your shoulders and down your arms and hands, feeling more and more energized. Moving down a little bit, beginning to stretch as energy comes up your throat. When it reaches your head and eyes, your eyes open naturally. You wake up, feeling refreshed and renewed, feeling relaxed.

Summary

The guided imagery above takes you through the sequential steps of any good imagery. First, you relax. Second, you "go to" a place that is comfortable and beautiful for you. By creating a special house or room to go to, you remind your subconscious that when you are there, work will be done. Each time you return you are able to go into deeper states of meditation. The screen has a special "safety" feature in this type of meditation. It allows you to step into it when you want to experience your images directly, and out of it when you want to observe rather than become involved. Finally, using the "bubble" helps you return to your natural state of consciousness in a gentle and easy fashion.

Use your creativity. Play with your visualizations. Make up stories of the perfect future and visualize/experience yourself in the story. The variations are endless and only limited by your imagination. So explore, enjoy, and have fun!

Eleven

Planes and Worlds of Consciousness

Imagine that you live in a seven-story building. In fact, you *own* the building! The building has so many rooms that you have not visited all of them. For most of your life, you have stayed on the ground floor—just to be near the earth. But even on the ground floor, you have not explored all the rooms. Once in a while, you have ventured up to the higher floors. From there you have looked down upon a different world than the one you can see from the ground. From the higher perspective, problems don't look as real, as serious, as they seem from the ground. It seems more peaceful on the higher floors, but you just have so much to do at ground level that you don't have a lot of time to hang around "up there." You visit occasionally, then hurry back to ground level.

This is the path of meditation. Meditation does not take you anywhere that you do not already own within your own mind. Meditation allows you to access the different planes and worlds of consciousness within the "building" of your own mind. Wouldn't it be nice to go anywhere in your building whenever you wished? Wouldn't it be nice to live on a higher floor for a while, and then return to your ground with new insights and new resolutions for old problems? The following is a "map," or guide to the building you own. It is offered in hopes that you will want to visit each floor for yourself. All you need do is go inside with your meditation, and visit the reality the map is directing you toward!

Ground Floor: The Physical Plane of Consciousness

Most of the world, most of the time, lives here on the physical plane of consciousness. On this plane, the physical body is very real to us. We devote great attention to keeping the body well, to keeping our house clean, to working for physical food and money. Yet even the physical has a component of energy that folks are just becoming aware of. We have a physical body and we also have an etheric or energy body, and both live on this first level, ground floor. Our physical body consists of organs, bones, and tissues. Our etheric body consists of mind/body energy that is often categorized by the chakra system. Chakra means "spinning wheel of energy." The next section will explore the chakras in detail. Knowing the relationship between their mind/body energy and the physical body is helpful to explain the work that we do while living on the ground floor.

The basic, or Root, chakra room is associated with Will energy, Universal Life. Here lies the Kundalini serpent of wisdom, waiting to rise into the higher realms. Here the physical organs of the kidneys and spinal column are nurtured. The second chakra, the Sacral room, is associated with physical plane force, animal life, and the sex organs. Energy in the Solar Plexus room, the third chakra, is associated with emotion, astral force and desire. It feeds the organs of the stomach, gall bladder, liver, and nervous system. In the Heart room we find the fourth chakra energy of life force and group consciousness. Here the physical organs of the heart, circulation, blood, and vagus nerve are nourished. The Throat room is the area of creative energy and physically associated with breathing and the alimentary canal. The Brow room, specifically the third eye center just above and between the eyebrows, nourishes our soul force and intuition while physically energizing the lower brain, left eye, nose, and upper portions of the nervous system. Finally, the Crown room, at the soft spot on the top of the head, represents our spiritual will and nourishes the upper brain and right eye. An excellent book on the interrelationship between energy, body, and planes of consciousness is *Chakras and Esoteric Healing* by Zachary F. Lansdowne, Ph.D.

Let's look at this material with respect to meditation. Meditation is a "vehicle" for traveling through our own consciousness, as well as a method for developing our awareness of our spiritual nature, our purpose, and our natural behaviors toward kindness and love. Obviously, it is very nice to live in the Sacral room of physical expression, but some people never come out of that room! They live for physical gratification, and without it their lives have no meaning. This room is closely aligned to the Solar Plexus room of emotion and desire. The desire may be broader than sex in the Solar Plexus room, expanding to desire for money, power, and influence. Desire to be the biggest, the best, to have the most, is within this room. It is a good place to visit, but I wouldn't want to live there all the time, because with desire, there is also disappointment, guilt, resentment, envy, and blame. Those emotions are not only not fun, but they are a breeding ground for physical health problems.

So how do we change rooms on the ground floor, the physical level? We change through meditation.

To move from the Solar Plexus room to the Heart room, center your meditations on positive regard. Meditate on love, on life, on healing. Rejoice in the good fortune of others. Be grateful for all that you have using the old adage, "count your blessings." Develop a Pollyanna outlook on life, refusing the negative and accepting wholeheartedly the positive. Use affirmations and loving kindness meditations.

Move to the Throat room of Creative energy by meditating on seed thoughts. "Seed" your consciousness with positive affirmations and powerful statements of your own creativity, your own value.

Move to the Brow room of Soul Force and Intuition through Mindfulness or Insight Meditation (see chapters 7 and 8). By becoming aware of our thoughts, we have the power to see beyond them into other aspects of our consciousness. We have the power to now explore other rooms of our building!

Second Floor: The Emotional Plane of Consciousness

The second floor houses our emotional body. Some refer to it as the astral or psychic plane. On this floor we explore our dreams, our fantasies, our fears, and our nightmares. It is the floor where good fights evil. Some believe it is the floor where ghosts hang around to complete unfinished business before they go higher in their own consciousness.

Why on Earth would we want to visit this floor? We visit to observe and release past "garbage" of our lives. If we have attained even a small level of mastery in our mindfulness meditation, we can visit here without danger. If we "know" that our thoughts are only thoughts, and that we can observe them without becoming involved in them, we can "watch the movies" that are always playing on the second floor. Many meditation traditions instruct new disciples to completely avoid this floor and go higher. Many "psychics" visit this floor and gain advice for their clients. Whether the advice is helpful or not depends upon the spiritual development of the psychic. If the psychic knows there is more to spirit than the astral plane, and knows how to guide their client beyond to higher planes, then the advice is felt by the client as warm and loving. However, if the person with proclaimed psychic abilities has not done their own spiritual homework, the advice is often fear-based, predicting dire consequences and outcomes or giving the client a list of things that he or she must do.

Treat this second floor of your consciousness as your personal movie theater. Go there in meditation to create beautiful images of your life. Watch the movies about the past and future with a sense of truly being in a movie theater, knowing that you can leave if the movie doesn't suit you, or watch it until the end if it is giving you good advice and insight.

Third Floor: The Mental Plane of Consciousness

On the third floor you house your Causal body or soul, and your Mental body or personality. Your Soul consists of your abstract thoughts, and directs you to the lessons you have chosen to learn while residing on the ground floor. These lessons appear the same for all of us and may be divided into three categories:

- Lessons about *Health*—how to use the higher qualities of love, will, and mind to overcome health issues.
- Lessons about *Wealth*—how to use the higher qualities of love, will, and mind to overcome issues about finances and material abundance.

- Lessons about *Happiness*—how to use the higher qualities of love, will, and mind to be in relationship in a positive way with ourselves and with others.

We are all studying these lessons. We are all taking tests arranged on the ground floor to see if we understand the curriculum that we have developed on the third floor. Just like when we were in school, sometimes the lessons are hard, and we have to do a lot of work before we "get it." Other times our understanding comes easily and we enjoy the lessons.

We use our personality (our concrete thoughts) to work through the lessons on the ground floor. We use our soul to guide us from the third floor. Soul guidance for ground floor lessons is always available. We just have to go to the third floor, through meditation, to find it.

Fourth Floor: The Buddhic Plane of Consciousness

Now, as we begin to go higher, the view of the ground begins to change. Imagine looking out a window on the ground floor of a building. Notice the trees, bushes, cars, and people. Now go up four stories and look at the same scene. The image changes. Now you are above the bushes and trees and cars and people. You are looking down upon what was once right before you. You have a different view, a different perspective.

The fourth floor contains the Buddhic notions of Spiritual Love and Spiritual Will. This Love and Will transcend the ground floor, personal ego ideal of love and will. Love at this level is Unconditional. It does not make demands for performance—such as, "I love you *if* you . . ." Will is more like the "Thy Will be done" kind, when you are looking for the highest outcome to all affairs.

Fifth Floor: The Atmic Plane of Consciousness

The hallmark of this floor is a unification of Will. Spiritual Will now manifests as "Father, My will is one with yours." There is a movement toward ultimate unity that begins on the fifth floor. No longer struggling between personal will and Spiritual Will, one realizes that there really is no difference.

Also beginning on this floor is a transcendence above and beyond words. An inner knowing, without word-images, comes into awareness. The "knowing" that you will be in the right place at the right time and take the right actions, all without personal effort. This beginning of unity is a truly freeing experience and is often found in moments of profound meditation.

Sixth Floor: The Monadic Plane of Consciousness

Here is the blending of Spiritual Will and Love with Wisdom and Active Intelligence. Here lies the knowing of oneness.

Once, my husband and I went on a meditative quest for "enlightenment." After many twists and turns in our venture, we were able to experience a moment (eternity) of oneness. During out visit to this sixth floor, we discovered that there was no difference between us and anything else. We were one with the trees, the grass, and the sky. There was no point where we ended and the world began. This was a "felt" experience, not an intellectual one. In that endless moment of eternity we were the vastness of all we beheld. We were One.

That kind of experience has not happened often to us. Visiting the sixth floor requires diligence, faith, and trust. It cannot be forced. We cannot barge our way in. But we can learn to relax and allow moments of oneness. We can intend to invite them into our lives through our meditation.

Seventh Floor: ADI Plane of Consciousness

Beyond words, beyond description, beyond thought, beyond feeling. The "great beyond" that is sometimes called the void or the "no-thing." A place of infinite healing as our separated self returns to its Source.

Back Home on the Ground

The final question is: why bother to visit all the rooms and floors in our house? Why not just live on the ground floor?

We visit because somewhere deep inside we know that we are more than flesh and bones. We know that there is something inside calling us to our purpose, our potential. We visit to discover that purpose and potential. We visit to receive deep healing and cleansing. We visit to transform our lives from the ordinary to the extraordinary. We visit because the building is ours, all the rooms are ours, and we are called to experience our fullness. Happy exploring!

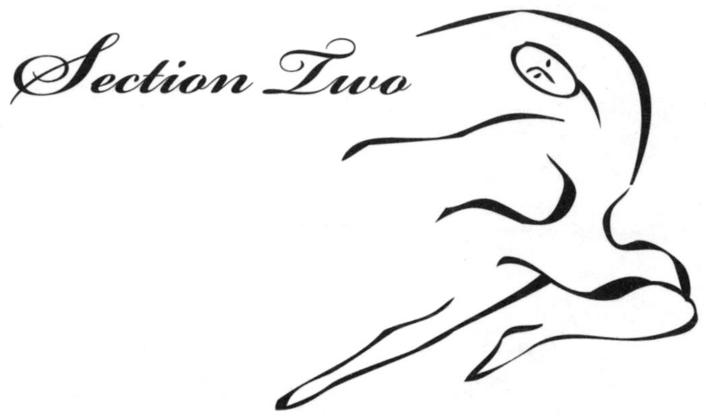

Section Two

Exploring the Energy of the Chakras

The material in this section is designed to inform and empower you based upon the ancient notion of chakra energy centers. *Chakra*, a Sanskrit term for "spinning wheel of energy," describes specific energy locations in the body/mind/spirit. These places, where finer energy infuses matter, contain the keys to our physical, mental, and spiritual Well Being.

One of the most valuable works you can do is to learn how to care for your chakra energy. In the coming chapters, we explore each chakra in depth and practice techniques for releasing negativity and inviting the full flow of chakra energy into our lives.

At the end of this section you will find a table that compares all seven chakras, and provides a summary and at-a-glance view of areas on which you may wish to focus your attention and energy.

Twelve

Overview of the Chakras

Chakra evolution can be traced from our ancestors to present day. The first chakra to develop fully was the root chakra. This energy system lies at the base of the spine and is concerned primarily with survival on the physical plane. Early cave dwellers had to use this energy to simply exist in a dangerous world. A single-minded focus on physical survival, security, health, money, and even death, reflects the activity of this primary energy. As physical needs were met, social relationships began to develop. Sensuality and sexuality between two people expanded to include pleasure and gratification available from others. Societies were built on the energy of the pelvic second chakra.

Once human beings had established safety and community, the personal power of the third chakra began developing in the solar plexus area. This is a masculine power of aggressiveness, competitiveness, recognition, status, self-image, and significance. Civilizations advanced and fell according to the dominating individual or ego involved. This chakra has been predominating through the middle of the twentieth century.

The "love-ins" of the 1960s, more than anything else, expressed the emergence of the fourth chakra, the heart. Opening of the heart chakra allows self-acceptance and generates feelings of love and caring for others as well as oneself.

This feminine center balances the self-preoccupation of the lower centers and acts as a bridge to higher emotions and energies.

As we begin our journey into the twenty-first century, the throat chakra has many of us literally choking! The opening of our creative abilities of self-expression is the next major lesson for many of us. This chakra of communication is seen in the growth of the Internet and World Wide Web. Instantaneous global communication challenges us to our highest levels of creativity and integration.

The brow chakra is the witness center, the joining of left and right brain wisdom and intelligence. The energies here connect us with our Higher Self and encourage the development and practical use of intuition.

Our spiritual center is located at the crown of the head and is our connection with cosmic consciousness. The energy here enables us to live in the moment, without desire; to be truly free of concerns, worries, doubts, and fears.

Exceptions to the Rule

Exceptions to the rule of chakra development have occurred throughout history. Jesus, Buddha, and other wise and holy men and women throughout the ages have demonstrated full mastery of all chakras. In fact, we all have access to all the power of our chakras at any given moment. We all have had experiences of unconditional love, of a sense of oneness with the beauty of our environment, of pure joy.

A Chakra Exercise

A simple exercise to begin enlivening your chakras is color imagery. Before going to sleep each night, take a couple of minutes to complete the following visualization. Begin by imaging a soft glow of red at the base of your spine. Notice the quality of the color and make it bright and beautiful. Now allow this red color to expand and flow up your body, down your arms and legs, and up into your head. Continue to allow red to expand through and out your body, surrounding you in a gentle red glow.

Repeat this process using the following colors and areas: orange in the pelvis, yellow in the solar plexus, green in the heart, blue in the throat, indigo at the brow, violet at the top of your head, and white surrounding your whole being. As you work with these colors, allow your breath to move the energy through and around you. Slow your breathing and let the colors flow and merge. Perform this exercise nightly and notice differences in feelings, sensations, and attitudes. This is one of the first steps you can take to begin to explore and balance the chakra energies within you.

Our purpose now is to learn how to fully use chakra energy for the highest good of our family, our community, the Earth, and us. This requires learning how to let go of negative emotions and conditions that disturb the flow of our energies, and learning how to refine and develop these energies for consistent positive manifestation in our world.

Thirteen

The Root Chakra and Basic Needs

The root chakra is located between the legs, its tip seating into the sacral-coccyx joint at the bottom of the tailbone. Called the *Muladhara* (support) chakra, it represents life, strength, power, and vitality. The energy to meet our basic needs resides here. This area is the key to grounding our dreams in the material world and in transforming etheric energy into observable reality. This is the universal life force, the Kundalini serpent of wisdom and life, lying coiled, ready to rise.

The goal of this first chakra is "mastery of the body so it can be used as a tool for Spirit" (from Alex Jones, *Seven Mansions of Color*). Only when we have firm control over our physical affairs, can we turn our attention outward in service.

Connected with the root chakra are the color red, the note C, the sound LAM, the element Earth, the Sun and the Moon. It is associated with the spinal column, adrenal glands, kidneys, rectum, legs, bones, feet, and the immune system. Caroline Myss, in the *Anatomy of Spirit,* refers to the root as the tribal chakra, and lists the primary strengths of this energy as tribal/family identity, bonding, tribal honor code, support and loyalty that give one a sense of safety and connection to the physical world. John Ruskin, in *Emotional Clearing,* identifies the primary feelings that indicate blocks in this chakra as threat of material loss, lack, bodily injury, disease, death, anxiety, possessiveness, selfishness, insecurity, limitation, delay, and desire for protection.

Psychological imbalance in the root chakra may manifest as role confusion, fear, martyrdom, anger, self-pressuring, greed, cruelty, and extreme impulsiveness.

Physical imbalance may manifest as anemia, iron deficiency, low blood pressure, decreased muscle tone, fatigue, and adrenal insufficiency.

Balanced, clear and bright, this basic energy provides affection, generosity, sensitivity to others, ambition to better one's self and strong physical propensities. Balancing the root results in the ability to take higher action to break mental conditioning and rapid change toward physical well-being.

Because this chakra contains old belief patterns that may still have authority in our lives, balancing it may require careful introspection. There is currently a series of commercials on television about medications "you just must have" to feel good. In each commercial, after listing all the benefits of the medication, a listing of its side effects are given. A commercial to lose weight says that side effects may include "an increased frequency of bowel movements, a urgent need to have them, and an inability to control them." Now, what is this commercial asking you to believe? That you can only lose weight if your GI system goes haywire! Beliefs about our body, our health, our money are deeply ingrained in us.

When we work with the root chakra, we work to change our beliefs about the very basic issues of our lives. We pledge to release beliefs that hinder us and we open to beliefs that fulfill our lives. Below are some guidelines to assist you in balancing this vital energy that supplies your basic needs.

Activities and Rituals

- Use the color red in your environment to stimulate will and life force, overcome depression and bring about positive change. Wear red, sit under a red light, look into a red painting, eat red-skinned fruits and vegetables (cherries, strawberries, radishes, beets, and tomatoes). Use your creativity to bring more red into your life!
- Listen to music written in the key of C, or sing songs in that key.

- Chant the sacred sound "LAM," to bring energy into the root chakra and open up the flow.
- Play with gemstones. The following is a partial listing of gemstones associated with the first chakra: garnet, ruby, coral, jasper, red tiger's eye, smoky quartz, obsidian, pyrite, and red agate. Place one of these stones in your pocket and, each time you touch it, affirm your physical vitality and material well-being. Sleep with a stone in your hand all night to allow your subconscious to affirm your willingness to accept improvement in all conditions associated with this chakra.
- Imagine traveling deep into the earth and planting there all your desires for material wellness. Release all fears and worries and use them as fertilizer for these new conditions that will manifest into your life. Perhaps you may wish to actually do just that! Write down all the beliefs you wish to release, then tear up the paper or burn it, saving the scraps or ashes. Now, write down all the desires you wish to manifest. Bury these desires in the ground, intact, and spread your "fertilizer" around them, for "out of the ashes rises the phoenix."

Summary

It is wise to attend to the energy of the root chakra when you are feeling "spacey" and out of sorts. When the plans you have made do not come to fruition, when you are feeling physically tired or ill, when you are constantly worried or fearful, then look to this energy at the base of your spine.

This chakra is particularly difficult for many of us. We have great ideas in our heads, but have a hard time grounding them in reality! We may be experiencing chronic health difficulties, chronic financial worries or other conditions that underlie our basic fears. Becoming aware of the energy of the root chakra, and using the activities listed in this chapter can help open up this vital earth energy. Pay particular attention to the mental attitudes and emotional feelings you may be holding onto in this area. Opening this chakra may be a simple as watching a movie that comforts you, or spending a day in nature, sitting under a tree. You know when you are balanced in the root chakra when you truly feel safe and secure. If you don't feel that way now, find small ways to bring these feelings into your life and then let them grow bigger and stronger. In Spirit, you are safe and secure, always. Now allow that feeling of Spirit to enter your daily affairs. Patience and practice will give you results!

Fourteen

The Pelvic Chakra and Relationships

The pelvic chakra is located just above the pubic bone on the front and back of the body. Its tip goes into the center of the sacrum. Called the *Svadisthana* (vital force) chakra, it represents optimism, self-confidence, enthusiasm, and courage. The social ray of service to mankind resides here. This area is the key to centering our emotions of sensuality and sexuality. This is the chakra of duality, yin/yang, and understanding the significance of opposites, especially ourselves in relation to society.

The goal of this second chakra is "performance of one's duties for God without a self-motive or attachment to the fruits of action" (an old Krishna teaching).

Connected with the pelvic chakra are the color orange, the note D, the sound VAM, the element Water, the Moon and the planet Venus. It is associated with the sexual organs, large intestine, lower vertebrae, pelvis, hip area, appendix, and bladder. In *Anatomy of Spirit,* Caroline Myss refers to it as the relationships chakra, and lists the primary strengths of this energy as the ability and stamina to survive financially and physically on one's own, to defend and protect oneself, to take risks, and the resilience to recover from loss. John Ruskin, in *Emotional Clearing,* identifies the primary feelings that indicate blocks in this chakra as sexual desire, frustration, compulsiveness, inhibition, cravings for touch, food, drink, smoking, drugs, entertainment, and luxury.

Psychological imbalance in the pelvic chakra may manifest as greed, abandonment, defensiveness, and self-consciousness.

Physical imbalance may manifest as sexual disorders, immune system dysfunction, muscle spasms, and weakness.

Balanced, clear and bright, this orange energy provides optimism, hospitality, and humanitarianism. Balancing the second chakra results in the ability to overcome suspicion, insecurity, and lack of trust and the power to follow good rules and overcome bad habits.

The pelvic chakra contains belief patterns associated with our sense of self, our sexuality, and our relationships to society. It is the chakra of attachments. Having developed to some extent a comfortable relationship with our own bodies, we now reach out to explore others. We become attached to our mate, our house, and our position in society. Any change disrupts our sense of self and we spend a lot of time avoiding all change. This avoidance dampens our creativity and our ability to go beyond our present conditions. The work of the pelvic chakra is about taking risks, taking charge of our lives. It is about choosing our companions wisely and gently allowing the negative to leave our lives. Remember that the element water is associated with this chakra. Discover in the pelvic chakra how to let go and flow. We detach from our addictions to food, drink, drugs . . . and from our addictions to people, places, and things. An affirmation I have found helpful and repeat often is: "I relax, I release, I let go, and I flow in the spirit of love."

Below are some guidelines to assist you in balancing this orange energy, which supplies your relationship needs.

Activities and Rituals

- Use the color orange in your environment to stimulate social enterprise and creativity. Orange is a social color and good in community centers, meeting places, areas of creative study, and hospital rooms. An orange wardrobe will fill you with feelings of courage and optimism. Eat orange-skinned fruits and vegetables (oranges, tangerines, carrots, etc.). Use your creativity to bring more orange into your life!

- Listen to music in the key of D, or simply hum this tone.
- Chant the sacred sound of "VAM" over and over, out loud, and let its vibration heal you.
- Play with gemstones. Carnelian is the most common gemstone associated with the second chakra. Place a carnelian stone in your pocket and each time you touch it, affirm your physical vitality and material well being. Sleep with a stone in your hand all night to allow your subconscious to affirm your willingness to accept improvement in all conditions associated with relationships and creativity.
- Imagine floating down a gentle river. Release all attachments by making them part of the passing landscape. You observe and you let go. Call to mind all things you think you must have to be happy, and let each go. If you have a moving body of water near you—a creek, stream or river, write down your attachments on a piece of environmentally friendly paper. Shape the paper into a boat and watch your attachments float away from your life.

Summary

Difficulties with relationships, with sensuality and sexuality, and resentment and blame of others indicate blocks in this chakra. This chakra is often closed by early negative experiences with groups. (Recall trying to be with the "in-crowd" in high school or experiencing difficulty on your first job?—again, the issue of fitting in.)

To open this chakra often requires acts of forgiveness. Use gentle meditations to release past hurts and resentments. Sometimes it requires a change of attitude about people and society. I like the model used by the Nature Conservancy. Instead of condemning society for the destruction of natural habitats, or organizing protests, the Nature Conservancy simply goes about quietly buying land. When they see land that is going to be used for a potentially harmful activity, they buy it. They don't use hate or anger. They quietly make a difference because they know that if they own the land, then they can use it to benefit nature and the Earth.

You, too, can quietly make a difference in your relationships. Change your attitude and accomplish your goals in a new way. This is the message of the second chakra.

Fifteen

The Solar Plexus Chakra and Personal Power

The tip of the solar plexus chakra seats directly into the diaphragm between thoracic vertebra T12 and lumbar vertebrae L1. Called the *Manipura* (jewel) chakra, it represents mental or intellectual power, happiness and joy. Sometimes referred to as the yellow Christ ray of wisdom, this area is the key to expressing our personal power. Our actions become motivated by the inspiration of vision and reason and are performed with the qualities of patience and self-control.

The goal of the third chakra is "control over the body and mind" (from Alex Jones' *Seven Mansions of Color*).

Connected with the solar plexus chakra are the color yellow, the note E, the sound RAM, the element Fire, and the planet Mercury. The solar plexus is associated with the stomach, liver, gall bladder, pancreas, spleen, and the nervous system. Caroline Myss, in *Anatomy of Spirit,* refers to the navel as the chakra of personal power and lists the primary strengths of this energy as self-esteem, self-respect, self-discipline, ambition, ability to generate action, ability to handle crisis, courage to take risks, generosity, ethics, and strength of character. John Ruskin, in *Emotional Clearing,* identifies the primary feelings that indicate blocks in this chakra as anger, aggressiveness, hostility, frustration, sense of worthlessness, inadequacy, helplessness, weakness, emptiness, feelings of being blocked, used, blamed, mistreated, and not getting the credit deserved.

Psychological imbalance in the naval chakra may manifest as worry, anxiety, and decreased mental sharpness.

Physical imbalance may manifest as digestive disorders, sinus and allergy problems, skin disorders, and blood sugar disorders.

Balanced, the solar plexus chakra provides an increased force of will, warmth, and the male energy to manifest. Balancing the third chakra results in high creativity, great precision and analytical abilities, flexibility and adaptability to change, efficiency in planning and organizing work and effectiveness in problem solving.

The solar plexus chakra contains belief patterns we hold about ourselves. It is the chakra of the personality or ego. In this chakra we typically experience the world as either "good for me" or "bad for me." Events and people who are good for me bring joy, those who are bad for me bring anger. The element Fire rules this chakra, and the fire of the ego is often felt here.

Another issue in this chakra is the issue of power. Many baby boomers have shied away from the notion of power. Power represented the establishment and injustice. It is now time to claim our true power—the power of Christ to heal and change the world. This power is not from the ego, but from higher guidance and wisdom. With true personal power we become leaders and world servers, and truly fulfill our missions here.

Below are some guidelines to assist you in developing an authentic personal power.

Activities and Rituals

- Write your personal mission statement (using yellow legal paper, of course!) First determine three action verbs that describe what you do. Use power words such as "empower, serve, extend, promote, etc."). Next list what these words apply to (healing, teaching, love, peace, etc.). And finally state who you are going to be with when you are performing your mission (friends, government, business, groups, etc.). Your mission statement must be bold enough to inspire you and broad enough to apply to all aspects of your life. After playing with words for months, I developed the following mission statement for myself. "My mission is to explore, facilitate, and advance well being in myself, in individuals, in groups and organizations." This statement applies to my own inner explorations and to my public roles as a polarity therapist, a storekeeper, a meditation instructor, and a professional educational consultant. I use it as my daily focus. For more information about mission statements, read *The Path* by Laurie Beth Jones.

- Use the color yellow in your environment to stimulate your joy of living. Yellow is the color of intellect and is good in libraries and study rooms. A yellow wardrobe will fill you with feelings of joy and security. Eat yellow-skinned fruits and vegetables (corn, squash, lemons, bananas, pineapples, grapefruit, melons, etc.).
- Listen to music in the key of E (not very common, I'll admit), so try humming in the key of E.
- Chant the sacred word RAM out loud to bring power to your center.
- Play with gemstones, especially yellow citrine, amber, gold tiger's eye, light smoky quartz and yellow jade. Place these stones in your pocket and each time you touch them, affirm your power to fulfill your mission and live your dreams. Sleep with a stone in your hand all night to allow your subconscious to affirm your willingness to accept genuine personal power in your life.
- Open up your power center by doing the following exercise adapted from Chi-Lel Chi Gong (see References section). Sit and place your hands in front of you, with your middle fingers on your navel (belly button). Now gently open your hands while imagining that you are releasing any energy that is holding you back into the universe. After slowly releasing for several seconds, reverse the motion and draw fresh universal energy back into you. Use your hands and mind in this way to release and renew. You may spend several minutes or several hours doing this technique. You may also use

this method to open and cleanse any chakra area by moving your hands to that area and repeating the process.

Summary

Our ability to make our way in this world, to be empowered to action, to reach our goals, lies in the solar plexus chakra. Misuse of this energy results in ego domination and domination over others. You know when the power is being misused when actions are motivated by anger, jealously, and fear. When you feel "better than" everyone else or look down on other people. Correct use results in having the ability to effect change for the better in our lives and the lives around us. The feeling of power comes from deep within—a power to do right. We are all powerful. Most of us do not know it. Opening and clearing the energy of the solar plexus enables us to use our power for the highest good of all concerned.

Sixteen

The Heart Chakra and Love & Healing

The heart chakra surrounds the area of the physical heart. Called the *Anahata* (unbeaten) chakra, it represents the emotional power of love. This area is the key to balance, harmony, peacemaking, hope, growth, healing, and love. Our actions become motivated by the quality of unconditional love, acceptance of self and others, and right use of compassion.

The goal of the fourth chakra is to "use the force of Love to bring about profound changes in ourselves and in our world" (from Alex Jones, *Seven Mansions of Color*).

Connected with the heart chakra are the color green, the note F, the sound YAM, the element Air, and the planet Jupiter. This energy is associated with the heart, circulatory system, ribs, breasts, thymus gland, lungs, vagus nerve, and the shoulders, arms, and upper back. Caroline Myss, in *Anatomy of Spirit,* refers to the heart as the chakra of emotional power and lists the primary strengths of this energy as love, forgiveness, compassion, dedication, inspiration, hope, trust, and the ability to heal oneself and others. John Ruskin, in *Emotional Clearing,* identifies the primary feelings that indicate blocks in the heart as loneliness, isolation, sadness, shame, jealousy, grief over loss, not being taken care of, not being accepted, being hated, or hating others.

Psychological imbalance in the heart chakra may manifest as crisis, mood swings, and general panic.

Physical imbalance may manifest as increase of heart rate, palpitation, arrhythmias, and panic attacks.

Balanced, the heart chakra provides generosity, nurturing, calming, relaxing, expanding, and strengthening of the heart. Balancing the fourth chakra results in feelings of brotherhood and sisterhood, prosperity, helpfulness, and unconditional love. These qualities help us to uplift others so they may also love and respect themselves.

The heart chakra contains belief patterns we hold about life itself. It is the chakra that teaches the lesson of forgiveness. Through the years we have learned to place emphasis on conditions for loving and being loved. Many of us grew up feeling "not good enough" and believing that if only we could do or be something else, we would be loved. With each action we asked: "If I do this for you, will you love me?" And with each disappointment we became bitter and resentful. Opening the heart chakra involves learning to love without dependency on external cause. Learning to love simply because we *are* love. Learning to forgive because we know that we are spirit and cannot be harmed. *A Course in Miracles* says: "I forgive you for what you did not do to me." In other words, "I know that as spirit, I cannot be harmed by you." That is a profound concept. Unconditional love means to accept others and ourselves without attachment, loving simply because that is what we naturally do. This is no easy task, and we all have daily opportunities to practice giving love. When a person is angry or hurting, they are asking for love. When we can give love regardless of their behavior, then we have practiced one of our major life lessons.

Below are some guidelines to assist you in developing an unconditional love.

Activities and Rituals

- Write out affirmations of love. Louise Hay has some great affirmation tapes available. My favorite is on *Songs of Affirmation* by Louise Hay and Joshua Leeds, and is called "All is Well." The lyrics go something like this:

"I love and accept myself exactly as I am . . . all is well in my world . . ." You see, if you love yourself and all is well, then nothing can bother you, there is nothing to forgive, and there is nothing to do but share your love with others.

- Another affirmation is a variation on the ancient Buddhist loving-kindness meditation. You begin by using the first person, *I,* and then progress to second person, *you,* and finally including *all.* "May (I, you, all) be filled with loving-kindness. May (I, you, all) be well. May (I, you, all) be peaceful and at ease. May (I, you, all) be happy."
- Listen to music written in the Key of F, or hum that note.
- Chant the sacred sound YAM out loud and often.
- Use the color green in your environment to stimulate healing, well being, and prosperity. Green promotes a sense of rest and relaxation and is good in bedrooms, hospital rooms, and meeting rooms where love is needed. A green wardrobe brings balance and harmony and fills you with feelings of serene, calming peace. Eat green fruits and vegetables including lettuce, green beans, broccoli, asparagus, green peas, spinach, limes, green apples, honey-dew melons, etc.
- Play with gemstones, especially emerald, peridot, tourmaline, jade, malachite, green calcite, aventurine, bloodstone, fluorite, and unakite. Place these stones in your pocket and each time you touch them, affirm your power to love unconditionally. Sleep with a stone in your hand all night to allow your subconscious to affirm your willingness to accept genuine love in your life.

Summary

Opening the heart to love may take a lifetime, or several. It is often easier for us to love our children, or our pets, more than it is to love ourselves. Yet the paradox is that we can only give others the love we feel inside.

As I stated earlier, most of us have the unloving feeling of "not being good enough" buried deep inside, of not being worthy of love from others, much less ourselves. Yet when we cannot love ourselves, we cannot truly love another. There is an excellent audiotape I often listen to by Roland D. Nadeau and Deborah Riegel called *I Am Worthy*. The tape is a series of affirmations spoken in both male and female voices designed to create a deep experience of worthiness. When we feel worthy of love, then we can share that love. And when we can share love with all beings, we have awakened the heart chakra to a wonderful new universe of love.

Seventeen

The Throat Chakra and Expression

The throat chakra is in the front and back of the throat area, its tip seats into the third cervical vertebrae. Called the *Vishuddhi* (pure) chakra, it represents the emotional power of expression. This area is the key to giving and receiving, and to speaking our truth. Our actions become motivated by the qualities of inspiration, creativity, spiritual understanding, faith, and devotion.

The goal of the fifth chakra is to "(establish) the kingdom of peace . . . in the soul as the once restless, sense-distracted mind is absorbed within to a state of tranquility" (Alex Jones, *Seven Mansions of Color*).

Connected with the throat chakra are the color blue, the note G, the sound HAM, the element Ether, and the planet Saturn. This energy is associated with the thyroid, bronchi, lungs, alimentary canal, neck vertebrae, mouth, jaw and teeth. Caroline Myss (in *Anatomy of Spirit*) refers to the throat as the power-of-will chakra, and lists the primary strengths of this energy as faith, self-knowledge, personal authority, and the capacity to make decisions. John Ruskin, in *Emotional Clearing*, identifies the primary feelings that indicate blocks in the throat as not being able to express yourself, inner emptiness resulting from intense creative work, being creatively blocked, or the desire to create or express.

Psychological imbalance in the throat chakra may manifest as fear of success, fear of power, and frustration.

Physical imbalance may manifest as respiratory or bronchial problems.

Balanced, the throat chakra provides the qualities of joy, relaxation, increased visualization, and communication. The channel between the heart and brow becomes open and flowing. Balancing the fifth chakra relieves over-reactions and aggressive impulses, impulse activity and jumping from one situation to another. "The body becomes immobile and the imagination, memory and understanding are no longer obstacles to the blessings received from God" (Alex Jones, *Seven Mansions of Color*).

The throat chakra contains encapsulated energy in the form of words and thoughts. Our ability to truly express ourselves becomes blocked by all the old words we cling to. As our vibrations rise in frequency, the throat chakra often forms a bottleneck of energy. Many of us who have successfully dealt with the first four chakras (more or less) become caught in our attempts to open this area. We feel the energy constriction by the chronic tension in our necks, the tightness in our shoulders and jaws. We experience all these thoughts constantly running through our meditations and we are amazed sometimes at what comes out of our mouths!

Clear expression requires inner silence, the ability to control the body, moods and habits at will and to speak clearly with a deep, spiritual understanding. Knowing that what we express outwardly returns to us, increased, the major lesson of the throat chakra is to express that which we want to receive. It seems sometimes that despite our best efforts, we continue to react to new situations in old ways, to express our past beliefs instead of our new understandings. The throat chakra is the vehicle for expression for all other chakras and is therefore connected to every detail of our lives. Old issues emerge here for us to take a look at and resolve. It challenges us to learn the nature of the power of choice.

Below are some guidelines to assist you in opening the expression of the throat.

Activities and Rituals

- Practice mindfulness meditation. Give yourself twenty minutes each day to sit quietly, feel your breath coming and going through your nostrils, and simply observe your thoughts. Become an impartial witness to your own mental activity. Learn to observe the encapsulated energy of thought and to free it by letting it go. By doing this daily, you will begin to experience the power of inner silence. From this inner silence you can express right action in each present moment.
- Listen to music in the key of G, or simply hum this tone.
- Chant the sacred sound of "HAM" over and over, out loud, and let its vibration heal you.
- Use the color blue in your environment to stimulate spiritual freedom and creativity. Blue relaxes the mind, is cooling, and can make a room seem larger. A blue wardrobe can bring a person in touch with his or her inner self and enables a calm and tranquil expression of ideas and information. Eat blue-skinned fruits and berries, potatoes, fish, and veal.
- Play with gemstones, especially turquoise, celestite, aquamarine, blue topaz, amazonite, blue agate, and dumortierite. Place these stones in your pocket and each time you touch them, affirm your choice to receive inner guidance and outward expression. Sleep with a stone in your hand all night to allow your subconscious to affirm your willingness to accept activation of your power of expression.

Summary

Working with the throat area allows us to become free of the past. How many times have you remembered words you said, or words said by others, that were not of benefit to the present moment? It seems as if we are constantly "talking" to ourselves—and many of the words are ones of judgment, resentment, guilt, and so forth. I recently spent several days mentally rehearsing a conversation I had with an extremely judgmental person. I thought about what I would say to her next, what I should have said then, and what I thought about her in general. In the meantime, the energy in my throat area became dense and clogged—with all those words and emotions. Through mindfulness meditation, it finally dawned on me that not only did I not want to continue this train of thinking, but also I really did not want to encounter this person in the future. It would be of no benefit to engage in another argument—to her or to me. As I began to release the need to "correct her," I also released the need to relive the conversation. Now, a week later, I can barely remember what was said. This is an important lesson for one who used to love a good argument, and who loved to win a point. It is truly healthier to release and forgive and, as a bumper sticker I once saw said: "Get over it!"

Eighteen

The Brow Chakra and Inner Wisdom

The brow chakra is located on the forehead and the back of the head, the tip seats into the center of the head. Called the *Ajna* (command) chakra, it represents the power of transcendence. This area is the key to balanced thinking and feeling. Our actions become more consistent, with increased wisdom, intuition, concentration, and increased sensitivity to subtle energy.

The goal of the sixth chakra is "to become aware of the cosmic manifestations of God/Goddess, All That Is, including love, wisdom, joy and light" (Alex Jones, from *Seven Mansions of Color*).

Connected with the brow chakra are the color indigo, the note A, the sound OM, the element energy, and the planet Uranus. This energy is associated with the pituitary and pineal glands, brain and neurological system, eyes, ears, and nose. In her *Anatomy of Spirit,* Carolyn Myss refers to the forehead or brow as the power-of-mind chakra, and lists the primary strengths of this energy as intellectual abilities and skills, evaluation of conscious and unconscious insights, receiving inspiration, generating great acts of creativity and intuitive reasoning. John Ruskin (in *Emotional Clearing*) identifies the primary feeling in the brow as transcendental consciousness of Higher Self. He states that: "We don't experience doing-to or being done-to, but just doing."

Psychological imbalance in the brow chakra may manifest as superiority, power addiction, and self-absorption.

Physical imbalance may manifest as dependency and substance abuse.

Balanced, the brow chakra provides the qualities of spiritual perception and intuition. Our consciousness is uplifted from preoccupation with the world of sensations, and we experience an awakened realization of other planes of existence and other valid realities.

The transcendence quality of the brow chakra manifests as a true transformation in our worldly outlook. Imagine living on the first floor of a large apartment building. When you look out the window, you see the world from a level plane. Cars still look like cars, and people look like people. You can rearrange the interior of your apartment again and again, but you are still looking out on the same world. Now imagine moving up to the thirty-fifth floor of the same building. You look outside and now you see everything differently. Cars no longer look like cars; they look like colorful, moving geometric shapes. People look like tiny moving elements of color. Your perspective has changed. You no longer see life in the same way. This is true transformation. It is an effortless experience of seeing all life with a broader perspective. No longer bound by thoughts and feelings from the past, we now have the ability to co-create our world from a higher level of consciousness. We are balanced within ourselves and within our multiple worlds of energy. From this point of true power, we are able to manifest things into the now at will. Unbound from space and time, we become masters of our own reality.

Below are some guidelines to assist you in opening the transcendence of the brow chakra.

Activities and Rituals

- Practice mantra meditation. The most basic and simple chant is to "sing" the word "OM." Sing "OOOOOOOOOMMMMMMM" over and over. Notice as you do that your breath becomes longer, that the sound becomes freer, that the tone changes to match your energy. Continue this for ten minutes without interruption, and you are well on your way to accessing transcendent energy. OM is the universal sound of this energy.

- Listen to music in the key of A, or simply hum this tone.
- Use the color indigo in your environment to call to you wisdom and intuition. Meditate on the color indigo and allow its energy to move through your being. Focus on the deep, blue-violet softness and richness of this color. Imagine moving down through the waters of the Gulf Stream, which are indigo in color. Move gently down and down until you become aware of a deep, inner peace, the merging of your consciousness with All That Is. Rest in this peace, without words. Allow transformation to occur of its own, naturally.
- Play with gemstones, especially sapphire, sodalite, and lapis lazuli. Place these stones in your pocket and each time you touch them, affirm your choice to effortlessly transcend the beliefs that bind you to the past. Sleep with a stone in your hand all night to allow your subconscious to affirm your willingness to live in the present moment.

Summary

The brow chakra holds many mysteries. I once met an Indian Swami or holy man. He wore a clay marking over his brow chakra, just above his eyes. I saw this man perform miracles of love, healing, and transformation. One day, someone asked him why he covered his brow chakra (third eye). Swamiji's answered something like this: "I cover my brow because the light of Spirit is greatest here. If you looked upon me without my cover, you would not see a person, you would only see light. Any if you only saw light, you would become afraid. I am here to guide you to love, not fear. And so I cover the light that is inside me. That same light is also in you, but you have not realized it yet." I never saw Swamiji without his "brow cover," so I cannot tell you that his words are true. I can tell you that I believe him.

Let your light shine in whatever way is comfortable for you. And know that that light is coming from your Higher Source, your True Self, from God/Goddess, all that is. We are here on this planet to "en-lighten," to heal, and to make whole.

Nineteen

The Crown Chakra and Oneness

The crown chakra is located on the top of the head, with its tip seated into the middle of the top of the head. Called the *Sahasrara* (thousand) chakra, it represents the experience of direct knowing. This area is the key to spiritual enlightenment. Included in its blessings are healing of the subtle body, calmness, gentleness, expansiveness, and harmony.

The goal of the seventh chakra is to "fulfill our purpose of existence by experiencing our oneness with the eternal now" (Alex Jones, *Seven Mansions of Color*).

Connected with the crown chakra are the color violet, the note B, the sound AUM, the element cosmic energy, and the planet Neptune. This energy is associated with the major body systems including the central nervous system, the muscular system, and the skin. Caroline Myss (in *Anatomy of Spirit*) refers to the crown as the spiritual connector chakra and lists the primary strengths of this energy as inner guidance, insight into healing, quality of trust beyond ordinary fears and devotion. John Ruskin (in *Emotional Clearing*) identifies the primary feeling in the brow as oneness with Self.

Psychological imbalance in the crown chakra may manifest as psychic attack, negativity, and paranoia.

Physical imbalances may manifest as insomnia, restlessness, and sensory dysfunctions.

Balanced, the crown chakra provides the qualities of divine realization, humility, and creative imagination. Our consciousness is uplifted beyond separation to the experience of oneness with all creation and the knowing that creation is nothing but our own selves.

Experience of the crown chakra energy cannot be explained in words. It is beyond duality and words can only point to the way. Most of us have had a brief experience of this blissful energy, whether we realized it at the time or not. In the mid-1980s, when my husband Charlie and I were becoming involved in our own spiritual development, we had just a moment of this energy. We were living in Augusta, Georgia, at the time and decided that we needed to become enlightened. We reasoned that a good place to become enlightened was in the mountains. So we rented a cabin for the weekend somewhere off the Blue Ridge Parkway. We arrived at night in dense fog, found the cabin and checked in, only to find that the restaurant was closed and there was no TV! When we woke up the next morning we discovered that our window looked out over a graveyard! Nevertheless, we went out looking for our enlightenment. We hiked down a gravel road looking for a waterfall. After several hours of hiking, and only finding horse droppings, we returned to the cabin and called it a day.

The second morning we decided to rent the horses that had obviously found the waterfall the day before. Neither one of us are experienced horse-riders, but Charlie was put on Spitfire and I was put on Fireball. The horses took off and we went bouncing along with them. Somewhere during that ride we both finally relaxed into the realization that the horses were totally out of control and that at any moment we would be thrown off to our deaths! Then it happened. We had given up control, and were allowed to experience Truth. For a moment, or an eternity, we could not tell which and it does not matter, we became one with All. There was no separation, no difference, between ourselves and the horses, the grass, the trees, the horizon, the earth, the sky. We were All That Is and All That Is was us. Just as suddenly as it began, the experience ended. We were back on the horses riding toward the barn. We dismounted, got in the car, checked out of the cabin, and came home. We had experienced what we intended; though not *how* we intended it. That, dear reader, is oneness. It has happened to you. It will happen again for all of us.

Below are some guidelines to assist you in opening to the oneness of the crown chakra.

Activities and Rituals

- Practice silent awareness of the vastness, the space, the infinite bliss found in nature.
- Intend to experience your Self and surrender to all of life.
- Listen to music in the key of B, or simply hum this tone.
- Chant the sacred sound of "AUM" over and over, out loud, and let its vibration heal you.
- Use the color violet in your meditation or contemplation rooms. Meditate on the color violet and white and allow its energy to move through your being.
- Play with gemstones, especially amethyst and clear quartz. Place a crystal on your nightstand to remind you of the pure Light of the infinite, eternal now.
- As Ram Dass says, simply "Be here now," living without desire each present moment.

Summary

Living in a state of oneness is very rare. Experiencing moments of oneness can be cultivated through meditation, nature, and even physical activity. Though I have never participated in extreme sports such as mountain climbing, parachuting, and marathons, I am convinced that the reward for these sports is that state of perfect flow, where the participant is truly *one* with the mountain, the sky, or the road.

As long as we feel enclosed within our bodies, we are separate. When our spirit expands outward to include our environment, we begin to sense feelings of belonging. When our spirits expand even further, we know that we are one with all, eternal and safe; healed and whole. This is the lesson of the crown chakra. It is a lesson we are all destined to learn!

Twenty

Rainbow of Lights

We conclude this section on chakras by providing a guided meditation. Read the following aloud into a tape recorder, then play it back to listen to it, or have a friend read it aloud to you, or simply read it over once, close your eyes, and remember the essence.

Chakra imagery is very healing and helpful. We have a group that meets weekly for meditation and inspiration. We always include some form of chakra energy imagery in each meditation we do. It is an easy and effective way to bring balance into your physical, mental, and energy body. Enjoy!

Begin by taking several deep and full breaths. Now relax and imagine a rainbow, all the colors vivid and bright.

Look at or imagine the color red. Focus completely on the color red and allow the red to enter your body, just at the base of your spine. This red is your root, or grounding, color of physical vitality and basic survival on the physical plane. Release any darkness or dullness, allowing all your fears to flow out the base of your spine, down into the earth. Imagine the color red becoming more brilliant, more beautiful. Allow this wonderful red to move through your entire body, from the top of your head to the tips of your toes—cleansing, revitalizing, and healing.

Focus your attention now on the color orange. Allow this light to enter your body, in the area of the pelvis. Orange is the color of your relationships with yourself, your friends, your colleagues, your community, and society. Allow all past disagreements to flow out of your body, down into the earth. Make this orange more beautiful, vibrant. See all relationships healing, becoming whole. Allow this feeling of peace and cooperation to flow through you and out into the world as the color orange fills your body from head to toe.

Visualize a happy yellow color. Allow this brilliant yellow to enter into your solar plexus, the area just below your ribs. Let its light outshine the darkness caused by constant ego demands. Allow the yellow light of true personal power to fill your solar plexus with its confidence and contentment. Know that you are good enough, bright enough, worthy enough to attain your needs and desires. Feel the clear, personal power of yellow moving now through your body and out into the world. You are the light!

Imagine a brilliant, emerald green color beginning to circulate in your heart area. This green is of healing and of unconditional love. Allow darkness associated with jealously, resentment, and anger to leave this area. Send the green into every cell in your body and love each cell, tissue, organ, and system. Tell your body that you love it and release it now from fear and worry. Tell your mind that love transcends all and that you now resolve to replace negativity and fear with love. Allow this brilliant emerald green to flow through your body and out into the world, healing and loving all that you encounter. You are love.

Imagine a brilliant blue light flowing in and through your throat. This is the color of communication. Make this little blue light bigger and brighter. Allow yourself to open the blue lines of communication, within and without. Listen for the voice of your Higher Self. Open now brilliant, blue lines of communication to that part that oversees your life and can guide you on the path of true love, and joy, and peace.

Imagine an indigo light in your forehead, between your eyes. Feel the presence of this deep color of wisdom and knowledge manifesting in your being. You can call upon this wisdom to assist you in making decisions, in determining the right action, and in following your destiny. Allow this indigo wisdom to flow through every cell and atom of your body, and outward into your environment, to comfort and enlighten those around you as you move steadily upon the path of your Soul.

The clear violet light of transformation now flows in through the top of your head. Transformation of illness into wellness, of sadness into joy, of failure into success, and of anger and resentment into love. Allow this violet now to flow through your entire being, circulating into any remaining dark areas, cleansing and renewing your entire being.

When you look at a rainbow you see all the colors in perfect balance. By closing your eyes slightly you can see the colors merging together and becoming surrounded by a pure white glow. This white light of spirit contains all colors and is indeed their Source. Your Source is Spirit, God, Goddess, All That Is. All of these colors are being supplied to you all the time. It is your choice as to how to use them. Commit now to renewing their brilliance each moment, each day.

Note: For an audio version of this chakra meditation, see our Ten-Minute Rainbow Tune-Up cassette in the References section. My husband and I recorded this "quick" version for busy people who wanted a daily practice, but only had ten minutes a day of spare time!

	Root (*Muladhara*—Support)	Pelvic (*Svadisthana*—Vital Force)	Solar Plexus (*Manipura*—Jewel)	Heart (*Anahatha*—Unbeaten)	Throat (*Visshudhi*—Pure)	Brow (*Ajna*—Command)	Crown (*Sahasrara*—Thousand)
Location	Between the legs, its tip seating into the sacral-coccyx joint.	Just above the pubic bone on front & back of the body, its tip goes into the center of the sacrum.	Solar plexus area on front and back of body, tip seats directly into diaphragmatic hinge, between thoracic vertebra T12 & lumbar vertebra L1.	Heart and chest area.	In front and back of the throat, tip seats into cervical vertebra C3.	On forehead and back of head, tip seats into center of the head.	Top of the head, tip seats into middle of top of head.
Keywords	Life, Strength, Power.	Optimism, Self-Confidence, Enthusiasm, Courage.	Mental Power, Happiness, and Joy.	Love, Balance, Peacemaking, Hope, Growth, and Healing.	Inspiration, Creativity, Spiritual Understanding.	Wisdom, Intuition, Concentration, Subtle Energy.	Expansiveness, Gentleness, Calmness, Harmony.
Action	Will to live and physical vitality, kinesthetic, proprioceptive, and tactile senses.	Center of emotions related to sensuality and sexuality.	Related to who we are and our own personal power.	Front aspect = love. Rear aspect = will.	Giving and receiving, speaking our truth.	Intuition; Front = conceptual understanding. Rear = carrying out our ideas.	Experience of direct knowing.
Goal	Mastery of the body so it may be used as a tool for spirit.	Performance of one's duties without attachment to fruits of action.	Control over body and mind.	To use the force of love for personal and societal change.	To establish the kingdom of peace and share it with others.	To balance our thoughts and feelings with higher insight and intuition.	To experience oneness with the eternal now.

Table 4. The Seven Major Chakra Centers

	Root (*Muladhara*—Support)	Pelvic (*Svadisthana*—Vital Force)	Solar Plexus (*Manipura*—Jewel)	Heart (*Anahatha*—Unbeaten)	Throat (*Visshudhi*—Pure)	Brow (*Ajna*—Command)	Crown (*Sahasrara*—Thousand)
Glands & Organs	Spinal column, adrenals, kidneys, rectum, legs, bones, feet.	Sexual organs, immune system.	Stomach, liver, gall bladder, pancreas, spleen, nervous system.	Heart, circulatory system, thymus, vagus nerve, upper back.	Thyroid, bronchi, lungs, alimentary canal.	Pituitary, lower brain, left eye, ears, nose, nervous system.	Upper brain, right eye.
Color	Red	Orange	Yellow	Green	Blue	Royal blue to indigo	Deep purple to light violet to clear
Sound	"LAM"	"VAM"	"RAM"	"YAM"	"HAM"	"OM"	"AUM"
Note	C	D	E	F	G	A	B
Element	Earth	Water	Fire	Air	Ether	Energy	Cosmic Energy
Planet	Sun/Moon	Moon/Venus	Mercury	Jupiter	Saturn	Uranus	Neptune

Table 4. The Seven Major Chakra Centers (continued)

	Root (*Muladhara*—Support)	Pelvic (*Svadisthana*—Vital Force)	Solar Plexus (*Manipura*—Jewel)	Heart (*Anahathi*—Unbeaten)	Throat (*Visshudha*—Pure)	Brow (*Ajna*—Command)	Crown (*Sahasrara*—Thousand)
Unbalanced (Psychological)	Role confusion, fear, martyrdom, anger, self-pressuring	Greed, abandonment, defensiveness, self-consciousness.	Worry, anger, anxiety, decreased intelligence.	Crisis, mood swings, panic.	Fear of success, power, frustration.	Superiority, power addiction, self-absorption.	Psychic attack, negativity, paranoia.
Unbalanced (Physical)	Anemia, iron deficiency, low blood pressure, decreased muscle tone, fatigue, adrenal insufficiency.	Decreased immune system, muscle spasms.	Digestive disorders, sinus and allergy, skin disorders, blood sugar.	Speeding heart rate, palpitation, arrthymias, panic attacks.	Respiratory, bronchial problems.	Substance abuse, dependency.	Insomnia, restlessness, sensory dysfunctions.
Balanced	Affection, generosity, sensitivity to others, physically strong, higher action to break mental conditioning, rapid change toward physical health.	Sexual energy, creative energy.	Increased force of will, warmth, male energy to manifest.	Generosity, nurturing, calming, relaxing and expanding, strengthening heart, prosperity.	Joy, relaxation, increased visualization, communication, opens channel between heart and brow.	Regularity, increased intuition, wisdom, concentration, eyesight, memory, meditation, increased sensitivity to subtle energy.	Increased spirituality, enlightenment, subtle body healing, increased feminine energy, calmness, gentleness, expansiveness, harmony.

Table 4. The Seven Major Chakra Centers (continued)

	Root (*Muladhara*—Support)	**Pelvic** (*Svadisthana*—Vital Force)	**Solar Plexus** (*Manipura*—Jewel)	**Heart** (*Anahathi*—Unbeaten)	**Throat** (*Visshudha*—Pure)	**Brow** (*Ajna*—Command)	**Crown** (*Sahasrara*—Thousand)
Balancing Activities (Using Color)	Wear red, sit under a red light, look into a red painting, eat red-skinned fruits and vegetables.	Wear orange, decorate study rooms, meeting places with orange color.	Wear yellow, sit under the sun, bring yellow flowers into your room.	Wear green, bring green plants into you home or business, eat green vegetables and fruits.	Wear blue and use the color blue in your environment. Blue relaxes the mind!	Use the color indigo in your environment to call wisdom and intuition to you.	Use the color violet in your meditation and contemplation rooms.
Balancing Activities (Playing with Gemstones)	Garnet, ruby, coral, jasper, red tiger's eye, smoky quartz, obsidian, pyrite, agate.	Carnelian, agate.	Yellow citrine, amber, light smoky quartz, yellow jade.	Emerald, peridot, tourmaline, jade, malachite, green calcite, aventurine, bloodstone, fluorite, unikite, rhodochrosite, coral, garnet.	Turquoise, clelestite, aquamarine, blue topaz, amazonite, blue agate, dumortierite.	Sapphire, sodalite, lapis lazuli.	Amethyst, clear quartz, milk quartz.
Balancing Activities (Using Your Imagination)	Imagine yourself traveling deep into the earth, releasing all fears into the dark, moist earth.	Imagine yourself floating down a gentle river. Release all attachments, float, observe, and let go.	Imagine lying on a beach in the sun. The warm rays of the sun shine down upon you, relaxing and healing!	Imagine a tiny spark of light deep in your heart area. Allow this light to grow, warming, healing. See it expand to warm and heal all around you.	Sit quietly and observe your breath coming and going from your nose and mouth. Just be with the breath, letting all else go, mindful of the breath.	Imagine moving down through the deep indigo waters of the Gulf Stream. Move gently down and down until you merge with deep peace.	Intend to experience your Self and surrender to all Life during meditation. Completely let go and *be*.

Table 4. The Seven Major Chakra Centers (continued)

Root (*Muladhara*—Support)	Pelvic (*Svadisthana*—Vital Force)	Solar Plexus (*Manipura*—Jewel)	Heart (*Anahathi*—Unbeaten)	Throat (*Visshudha*—Pure)	Brow (*Ajna*—Command)	Crown (*Sahasrara*—Thousand)
Balancing Activities (Using Rituals)						
Write down all your fears, then burn the paper—saving the ashes. Now write down your desires and bury them, spreading the ashes to fertilize your desires.	Write down your attachments on a piece of biodegradable paper, shape them into a boat, and place the boat in a moving stream of water. Watch and let go!	Write out your personal mission statement (on yellow legal paper!) and post it on yellow notes everywhere! Remind yourself why you are here!	Write out affirmations of love, such as "I love and accept myself" or "May all beings be filled with loving-kindness." Repeat loving affirmations often.	Sleep with a blue stone in your hand one night (see gemstone list above). This allows your subconscious to activate your power of expression.	Practice mantra meditation. "Sing" the word Om, "OOMMM." Notice as you do that your breath becomes longer, the sound becomes more free, and you feel more relaxed.	Practice silent awareness of the vastness, the space, the infinite bliss found in nature. Surrender to the moment, as Ram Dass says, "Be Here Now."

Table 4. The Seven Major Chakra Centers (continued)

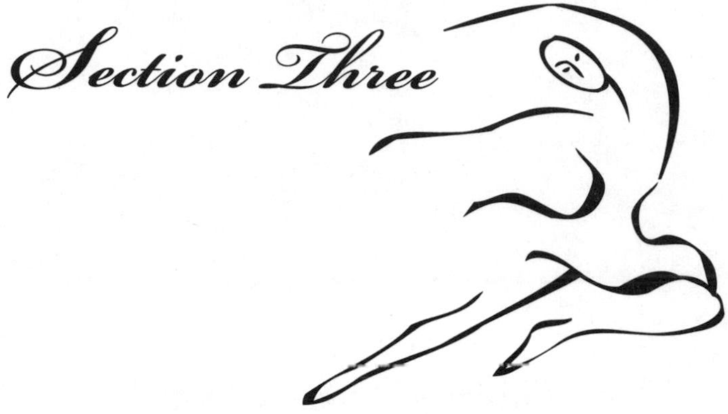

Polarity Energy, the Five Elements, and You

You will find here the concepts and tools you need to begin to follow the flow of elemental energy through your mind and body. This section contains basic information about Polarity Energy Balancing. The source of much of this information comes from my training as a Certified Associate Polarity Practitioner. Professional training to practice Polarity Therapy is available through instructors certified by the American Polarity Therapy Association (see "References and Resources, page 212).

It is not the intent to "train" polarity practitioners in this book. It is my intent, however, to use Polarity as a new way to view energy and healing. To begin, complete Table 5, the Polarity Self-Assessment, on page 125. Check all the boxes that apply and add your total score. Keep in mind your highest score as you read the chapters and find ways to balance any unbalanced areas in your body/mind/spirit. Most of all, experiment with the suggested activities and enjoy.

Twenty-one

Introduction to Mind-Body Types

Who are you? Of course, you are Spirit—eternal, infinite, and universal. When Spirit enters a body, the energy becomes denser as it binds itself to the earth plane. The Energy of Spirit appears as streams of consciousness. The ancients called them: Ether, Air, Fire, Water, and Earth. One or more of these streams (elements) dominate in us today.

Think about the last time you were with a group, and see if you can recognize each element in action. Sue sat quietly, observing, above it all. Someone called her spacey. Her ether element was strong! Joe was quick and alert. He came up with lots of ideas. A great inspiration to others, but most of the time he was just full of Air. Jack was a go-getter, risk taker, and liked being boss. He suggested many creative projects. Sometimes quick tempered, direct, and aggressive, Jack burned with the Fire of inner creativity. Mary used her deep, intuitive, emotional senses to tell everyone how she, and they, felt. Her Water element focused on the emotions of the group. Sam came up with practical ways to accomplish all the ideas of others. He was solid, dependable and down to earth. We need all five of these personalities blended and in balance, in order to accomplish our goals in life.

Overview

Polarity Therapy, developed by Dr. Randolph Stone, D.C., D.O. (1890–1981), is a comprehensive system of balancing these body/mind/spirit energies through hands on energy balancing, nutrition, exercise, and counseling.

According to Dr. Stone, the soul or spirit, as a unit, receives its fine energy from an Inner Source or Sun. Matter is the pole at the most remote distance away from the Source of energy. As the vibrations of energy slow down, they crystallize, producing matter. Mind is the mediator of function between spirit and matter. Mind is healthy and functioning properly when it is ruled by the soul or spirit. But when mind is ruled by the senses, then matter predominates and peace leaves.

The five elements of Polarity Therapy (Ether, Air, Fire, Water, Earth) are present in everything that exists on the earth plane. Everything is created from them. The difference in life forms is the difference of which element is predominant. In plants, the water element is predominant. Insects and snakes have two predominant elements, birds have three, and animals have four. Only in human beings are all five elements predominant. This fifth element, Ether, represents the choice of right and wrong. It allows the spiritual chakras to open and provide access to Higher realization. Each of the elements is represented in the lower 5 chakras and have the other four elements in them. For example, 50 percent of Ether is Ether and the other 50 percent is divided among the other four elements. The same ratios hold true for each of the lower five chakras. Dr. Stone explained that there is constant change on the physical plane because the relationship of the five elements is constantly shifting. The elements originate on the causal plane—they are subtle mind energy. But the elements are unstable because they are antagonistic to each other. This instability creates change; the cycles in life, day and night, the seasons, the stages of life, ups and downs, creation and expansion, crystallization and death. It is only upon the death of the physical body that the elements return to their own essence.

In terms of polarity, if we resist the changing cycles of life, we get out of balance and experience pain and dis-ease.

The Five Elements and Your Mind-Body Type

Ether is the prime element latent in all things, providing space and balance for all elements to unfold. Ether is essential to our sense of connectedness with spirit and well being. In the body, ether is space, particularly in the chest and joints. Out of balance, we have problems with our breathing, joint pain, and difficulties expressing ourselves. Balanced ether promotes our sense of joy and union. Lack of ether is connected with the feeling of grief and separateness.

AIR is lightness and movement. On a still day we feel listless and heavy, while on a windy day we feel refreshed and enlivened. Air is associated with the east, a new day, and new beginnings. Air signs include: Gemini (shoulders and arms, lungs and respiration); Libra (kidneys); Aquarius (legs). Imbalances are seen as nervous exhaustion, panic attacks, headaches, gas, bronchitis, heart problems, neuralgia, and leg cramps. Balanced air promotes our sense of love, devotion, and compassion.

Fire is light and heat. Fire is transformative and is associated with willpower and creative force. Fire is connected with the south, the summer, and purification. Fire signs include: Aries (head); Leo (solar plexus); Sagittarius (thighs). Fire imbalances include headaches, eye disorders, digestive disorders, liver problems, pain and weakness of the legs. Too much fire results in sympathetic dominance or the typical type A personality—stressed and burned-out! Unbalanced Fire shows as anger and resentment. Well-balanced fire is forgiveness and enthusiasm.

Water is the source of all life, formless and flowing. Water is associated with the west, the fall, the time to go deep and let our emotions flow. Water signs include: Cancer (breasts); Scorpio (genitals), and Pisces (feet). Imbalances show as breast tenderness and lumps, skin, menstrual, prostate problems and foot and back pain. Balanced water allows us to relax and let go, while unbalance reflects our attachment to worldly things.

Earth is dense, passive, the great provider. It has permanency and stability. Earth is associated with the north, winter, and material affairs. Earth signs include: Taurus (neck); Virgo (bowels); and Capricorn (knees). Balanced earth reflects in strong bones, active assimilation and elimination, and flexible necks.

When unbalanced, fear takes over and we experience neck stiffness, constipation and weak bones (osteoporosis). Balanced we find courage and contentment.

Self-Healing Activities

Use your imagination to bring elements into balance. To cool a "hot head," imagine floating in water. Generate new ideas by letting them soar in the clouds and then ground them by planting idea seeds deep in the earth.

Use your hands. Your right hand is your positive, or giving, hand. Your left hand is your negative, or receiving, hand. By placing your hands on your body opposite each other (front to back, side to side, or top to bottom) you automatically establish an energy flow between the positive and negative poles. Place your right hand over areas of tension or pain, areas that "feel" congested. Then place your left hand at a point a comfortable distance from your right, either above, to the side of, or behind your right hand. Just relax your hands on your body and you may sense the energy release as it flows from your right hand to your left. For example, if you have a sinus headache, place your right hand on your forehead and your left hand on your tummy. Relax and let the energy flow.

Place your left hand over "empty" areas of chronic tension. Place your right hand opposite (top to bottom, front to back or side to side). Now energy will flow to your left hand and the empty area from your right hand. For example, if you have chronic shoulder tightness, place your left hand on your shoulder and your right hand on your tummy. Relax and allow the energy to flow from your tummy to your shoulders.

Ether	Air	Fire	Water	Earth
Birth Date/Sign	☐ Gemini: 5/22–6/21	☐ Aries: 3/21–4/20	☐ Cancer: 6/22–7/21	☐ Taurus: 4/21–5/21
	☐ Libra: 9/21–10/23	☐ Leo: 7/24–8/23	☐ Scorpio: 10/24–11/22	☐ Virgo: 8/14–9/23
	☐ Aquarius: 1/21–2/19	☐ Sagittarius: 11/23–12/21	☐ Pisces: 2/20–3/20	☐ Capricorn: 12/22–1/20
☐ Sinus congestion	☐ Shallow breathing	☐ Sleep disturbances	☐ Breast lumps or tenderness	☐ Osteoporosis
☐ Breathing difficulties	☐ Tension in chest, locked scapulae	☐ Immune system difficulties	☐ Herpes	☐ Diarrhea
☐ Abdominal problems	☐ Heart problems	☐ Stomach ulcers	☐ Menstrual problems	☐ Constipation
☐ Joint problems	☐ Shoulder and/or arm problems	☐ Liver problems	☐ Prostate problems	☐ Colitis
☐ Throat problems	☐ All nervous system problems	☐ Digestive problems	☐ Foot problems	☐ Spastic colon
☐ Inability to express oneself	☐ Gas in abdominal area, flatulence and bloating	☐ Skin problems including rashes, spots, and acne	☐ Pelvic and lower back problems	☐ Hemorrhoids
☐ Hearing problems or hearing loss, including tinnitis	☐ Pain, especially headaches, neck pain, and muscle spasms	☐ Smoking or drinking alcohol	☐ Skin problems (with Fire element)	☐ Chronic tension in the neck, abdomen, or knees
	☐ Exhaustion	☐ Migraine headaches	☐ Overly sensitive to touch	
	☐ Arms feel numb	☐ Eye problems and disturbed vision	☐ Allergies	
	☐ Radiating pain (neuralgia)	☐ Overly anxious or constantly worried		

Total Each Column Below

☐ **Ether** ☐ **Air** ☐ **Fire** ☐ **Water** ☐ **Earth**

TABLE 5. POLARITY ENERGY SELF-ASSESSMENT

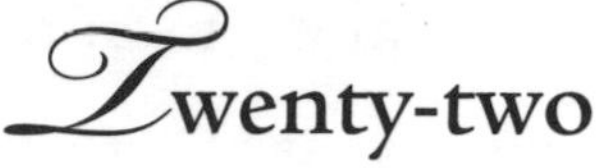

Twenty-two

Ether

The Ether element is the ground or field from which all other elements arise. Dr. Stone describes it as the "one river from which the other four rivers arise." Least dense of all the elements, Ether creates a unified field of subtle space for the movement of the other elements. The basic qualities of Ether are stillness, harmony and balance. It is the closest element in quality to the neutral center, or Source, and is the ground for manifestation of the mind-body complex. Its chakra center is located at the throat and the neuter field of the neck is a manifestation of it.

In essence, Ether is the space where everything happens. A person who feels "pressured by time" has their Ether out of balance. Ether in balance allows you to do everything with ease and without a sense of rushing or crowding.

Ether and the Emotions

Ether governs the mind and emotions and combines with other elements to create various qualities of emotion. Ether combines with itself in the Throat chakra, governing communication and the emotion of grief (ether in ether). As other elements interact with Ether, other emotions evolve in the lower chakras. Desire, in the heart chakra, represents a mixing of Air in Ether. Anger in the solar plexus is a combination of Ether and Fire. Lust in the pelvic area is Ether and Water, while Fear, located in the rectal area, is Earth in Ether.

Ether and the Body

In Polarity, every joint is a neuter point of harmony, balance, a sense of going back to the source. Energy crosses over every joint, providing the space for movement. Ether also provides the space for movement within all body cavities and even within the body cells themselves. All body functions require space in which to perform. A tightening of space signifies lack of Ether, while a feeling of "spaciness" indicates too much predominance of Ether with respect to other elements.

Ether and Dis-Ease

The medical profession currently diagnoses a disease by placing a label on a complex set of physical signs and symptoms. This label "encapsulates" the problem and places it in a category in which mechanical and chemical means may be used to resolve the problem. Polarity Therapy recognizes areas of dis-ease, areas where energy is not flowing smoothly. Dr. Stone stated: "Causes are always in the Energy Field, never in Matter." Lack of flow in the energy field may well invite dis-ease, however, it is a simple matter to encourage the energy to return to its natural, healthy state of flow. With this in mind, I now list potential dis-ease associated with the Ether element.

The problems listed in the following areas may indicate an imbalance of the Ether energies:

- Sinus congestion
- Breathing difficulties
- Abdominal problems
- Joint problems
- Throat problems

- Inability to express oneself
- Hearing problems, including ringing in the ears (tinnitis) and hearing loss

Balancing Ether

Ether is the most essential, purest, most perfect element latent in all things. It is non-tangible, the fundamental space out of which all other elements occur. So how does one go about balancing this elusive element?

First, remember the energy in your hands as described in the last Chapter. Your thumbs are Ether energy (as well as your big toes). To encourage the flow of ether over a particular joint, place the thumb of your right hand below the joint and the middle finger of your left hand above the joint. Gently allow the energy to flow between thumb and middle finger. You may also activate Ether energy by making a fist with one hand and gently holding the thumb of your other hand inside. This sends energy to balance Ether, the spleen and stomach, and worry.

If you are feeling particularly "spacey," as if there is too much energy in your head and none moving down below, try the following.

Place your right palm on the top of your head, then 1) Place your left index finger between your eyebrows and "connect the energy," feeling it begin to flow downward; 2) Move your left index finger to the tip of your nose and connect the energy; 3) Place all your left fingertips on the middle of your sternum and massage gently—feel the energy moving downward; 4) Move your left hand to the base of the sternum and hold gently directly over the solar plexus; finally, 5) Place your left fingertips over the top of the pubic bone. Steps 1–5 are performed while holding your right palm on the top of your head. Finally, 6) Leave your left hand on the top of your pubic bone and move the right hand from the top of your head to the base of your spine at the coccyx. Hold both positions gently until your feel the flow of energy going down your legs and out your feet.

If you want to run the Ether energy up instead of down, use the "Space Button." "Sit" on your left hand by placing your left fingertips at the junction between the coccyx and the sacrum, the hard bony area at the base of the lower back. Place two fingertips of your right hand on the "moustache area" between the upper lip and nose. Massage gently with the two upper fingers and then hold. Breathe deeply, and imagine a movement of energy up the back and over the top of your head to the "moustache area." Stop when you feel complete.

Summary

Balanced ether results in a "return to spirit." And a return to spirit balances ether. Any meditative techniques will work well for this balance. Periods of quiet in which you follow your own energy back into the quiet core of your being will open and expand the Ether element in your body. Body follows mind. Think space . . . Think balance . . . Think stillness . . . Think harmony. And after thinking them, feel them. Feel space . . . Feel balance . . . Feel stillness . . . Feel harmony. Feel your way into the spaciousness of Ether.

Twenty-three

Air

Air is wind and associated with movement. Located in the heart chakra, Air reflects our lightness and ease of movement. Like the wind, Air is pervasive and only perceptible when it moves. Like the wind, Air is changeable. On a still day we feel listless and heavy, while on a windy day we feel refreshed and enlivened. Air is the medium for carrying things. Externally it carries seeds, birds, sounds, while internally it carries energy and motion. The Air element is associated with the East—manifestation, dawning of the day, new beginnings and things coming into being. Air is movement and life!

In essence, Air is the movement of all things within the space of Ether. A person who feels that they have to rush around all the time, have to move quickly, has their Air out of balance. Air in balance allows free and relaxed motion, a sense of ease and flow.

Air and Movement

Air is associated with the five forms of movement in the body. Speed reflects Air in Air. A person who can't slow down, or one who can't speed up, or is scattered reflects Air in Air imbalance. Stretching is Ether in Air. One may "stretch" either physically or mentally! Shaking is Fire in Air. Trembling, uncertainty, indecisiveness indicate a need for grounding. Flowing reflects Water in Air. A sense of all movement flowing, all words in rhythm and harmony, a mental flow. Contracting is Earth in Air. Too much earth may manifest as a tightening, a closing off on every level.

Air and the Body

Air has its positive pole in the shoulders, ruled by Gemini, its neutral pole in the kidneys and adrenals, ruled by Libra, and its negative pole in the calves and ankles, ruled by Aquarius. The shoulders have been called the "wings of life." When the shoulders are rigid and tight, the Air element is congested in its positive pole, not flowing downward. Air also governs three major body systems—the respiratory system, the nervous system and the circulatory system. In my practice of Polarity Therapy, Air is the most common element to be out of balance. We stop "circulating." Stress stimulates the adrenals and simultaneously tenses the shoulders. Our energy becomes locked in the upper body and we are unable to ground and flow.

Air and Dis-Ease

Problems in the following areas may indicate an imbalance of the Air energies:

- Shallow breathing
- Tension in the chest, locked scapulae (shoulder blades)
- Heart problems
- Shoulder and/or arm problems
- All nervous system problems
- Gas in the abdominal area (flatulence and bloating)
- Pain, especially headaches, neck pain, and muscle spasm
- Exhaustion

- Arms feel numb
- Radiating pain (neuralgias)

Balancing Air

The Air element is associated with the negative (receiving) energy of the index finger and second toe. A very simple way to encourage the flow of Air is to massage these digits. A friend of mind was experiencing some of the dis-ease listed above and called me on the phone. I asked her to check out her second toe on both feet. "Wow" she said when she returned to the phone. "My right second toe is flexible, but my left is like concrete–it's really solid!" Needless to say, she was experiencing most of her dis-ease on the left side of her body. She began a diligent program of toe massage and the symptoms cleared. Dr. Stone insisted that the sign of healthy airflow was the ability to "pop" your second toe (i.e., pull gently on your toe and hear/feel the pop of joints releasing).

An excellent exercise to mobilize the flow of Air in the shoulder area is called the "Cliffhanger." Stand with your back to a sturdy table, countertop, or back of a chair. Place the heels of your hands slightly behind you on the supporting surface. Now gently slide your bottom straight down towards the floor, allowing your hands to receive the weight of your body. Feel your shoulder blades stretching and moving closer together. Maintain this position without strain for several seconds, and then slowly stand up. This exercise is great to do hourly if you work at a desk or computer.

Remember the polarity of your hands from chapter 21. Your left hand is a negative (receptive) charge, while your right hand is a positive (giving) charge. You can connect the poles of Air on your body simply by using your hands. Place one hand on your shoulder and the other hand on your low back/kidney area. Gently massage your shoulder and feel the energy begin to open and flow between shoulder and low back. Now move one hand down to your calf, while keeping the other on your low back. Massage your calf area and feel the energy flowing between calf and low back. To flow energy downward, use your left hand as the "bottom" one, keeping it closer to your feet than your right hand. To flow energy upward, use your left hand at the "top," keeping it closer to your head than your right hand. (Remember, energy flows from positive to negative, from your "positive, giving right hand to your negative, receiving left hand.)

Summary

Balanced Air allows you to open up the heart chakra and flow with the universal force of love in your life. With shoulders relaxed, breath deep, and heart open, you can meet any circumstance with flexibility. Change occurs. It really does! When we meet change with resistance and fear, we contract and temporarily lose this wonderful movement of Air. Relax and greet the winds of change in your life. They are bringing you movement and growth.

Twenty-four

Fire

Fire is light, heat, the Sun. Fire can flare up and get easily out of control. We speak of a "trial by fire" as a cleansing and growing experience. Fire has the quality of transformation. Associated with the third chakra, the solar plexus, Fire is the element of personal power, of will power. Fire under control can provide heat, warmth, and protection. Fire is the third "river of energy" which flows throughout body/mind. Its strength (or weakness) affects all other elements in powerful ways.

In essence, Fire is the heat and light of all things. A "fiery" person gets things done, but often at the cost of harmony. Fire in balance is the power to accomplish our will in our lives.

Fire and Metabolism

Fire is associated with the five aspects of metabolism in the body. Hunger is Fire in Fire. A fire in the belly, a hunger for the truth. Sleep is Ether in Fire. Too little Ether will provide no space for Fire to burn. This results in either sleeping too much or not being able to sleep at all. Thirst is Air in Fire. A thirst for knowledge, for information. Glow refers to the luster on the skin and represents Water in Fire. A healthy person has a bioluminescence, a quality of the skin that is absent in illness. Laziness, Earth in Fire, is literally doing nothing because the Fire has been buried.

Fire and the Body

Fire has its positive pole in the head, ruled by Aries, its neutral pole in the solar plexus, ruled by Leo, and its negative pole in the thighs, ruled by Sagittarius. Headstrong people are usually fiery in nature. The intense, overbearing, demanding, perfectionist reflects fire in the head. Anger and resentment, usually expressed in the form of ulcers, is too much fire in the belly. The liver is also considered an organ of Fire. Problems with the liver may be seen in vision problems. Leg weakness often reflects a lack of downward flow of Fire–its all stuck up in the belly and repressed there. Fire circulating freely permits us to move through life in a positive and exciting way.

Fire and Dis-Ease

Problems in the following areas may indicate an imbalance of the Fire energies:

- Sleep disturbances
- Immune system difficulties
- Stomach ulcers
- Liver problems
- Digestive problems
- Skin problems, including rashes, spots, and acne
- Smoking or drinking alcohol
- Migraine headaches
- Eye problems and disturbed vision
- Overanxious or constantly worried

Balancing Fire

The Fire element is associated with the positive (giving) energy of the middle finger and third toe. A very simple way to encourage the flow of Fire is to massage these digits. However, most of us have too much Fire. Just look at a person who uses the middle finger in a gesture of anger! This is repressed, and expressed Fire in action. In this case, Fire must be calmed rather than stimulated. Massaging the ring finger (the Water finger) will literally "put water on fire" to calm it down.

Fire is often suppressed in the belly area. We do not have a lot of opportunity to express this expansive energy. When angry, we cannot run around, scream and shout. (Our bosses or our families simply won't put up with it.) And we often cannot express Fire in a positive way, that is, by "shouting for joy" or performing vigorous exercise. You may find the following mental imagery useful for facilitating the flow of the current of Fire within you. It is called the Path of Fire.

The Fire element flows through a definite pathway within and around your body. Imagining this flow actually helps it move. As you perform the following imagery, note places where the Fire seems easy to imagine, and areas where it seems more difficult. The difficult areas indicate blocks that will resolve with gentle encouragement. Visualize a stream of energy coming in through the bottom of your left foot. Run this energy up your left leg and let it cross over from the left hip to the navel (belly button) area. From the navel, take this energy up to the right shoulder, across the shoulder and up the neck to your right ear. Let the energy cross over the top of your head and come down to the left ear. Now guide the energy down your neck and into your left shoulder. From here, take it down to your navel and across to your right hip. Now let the energy flow down your right leg and out the bottom of your right foot.

The majority of people who perform this exercise notice a definite resistance to the downward flow of energy. It is easier to bring the energy up and into the head than it is to allow the energy to flow down and out the right foot. This is reflective of our inability to "let go." We take in and hold on tight! One client with sinus problems, couldn't initially get the energy into the head. The flow went directly across the shoulders, thus cutting off the head entirely! With practice, the client was able to visualize the flow up over the head and down, and the sinus problems were greatly relieved.

Remember the polarity of your hands from chapter 21. Your left hand is a negative (receptive) charge, while your right hand is a positive (giving) charge. You can connect the poles of Fire on your body simply by using your hands. Place one hand on your head (the area of the eyes and forehead is especially effective) and the other hand on your solar plexus/belly area. Gently massage your belly and feel the energy begin to open and flow between it and your head. Now move one hand down to your thigh, while keeping the other on your belly. Massage your thigh and feel the energy flowing between thigh and belly. To flow energy downward, use your left hand as the "bottom" one, keeping it closer to your feet than your right hand. To flow energy upward, use your left hand at the "top," keeping it closer to your head than your right hand. (Remember, energy flows from positive to negative, from your "positive," or giving right hand to your "negative," or receiving left hand.)

Summary

Balanced Fire brings energy and vitality to life. It allows the action necessary for you to carry out your will. Fire brings a "spark" to your projects and relationships. It brings a "twinkle" to your eyes and a sense of excitement to your life. Fire under control provides protection and comfort. May you always have the fire of life burning brightly.

Twenty-five

Water

Water is formless, feminine, magical and healing. The moon influences its tides. The source of life, (we begin in water in the womb). Water is associated with purification and baptism. Depth of feeling, emotions and the ability to let them flow are a part of Water. A shape changer, Water exists in different forms under different conditions. Water needs the help from other elements to move, and is contained in and channels through other elements. Water is also a universal solvent, with abilities to dissolve materials. Located in the second chakra, Water is associated with our relationships with others and ourselves.

In essence, Water is versatile and adaptable. It has the ability to change in response to varying conditions. A person with the Water element dominant will "go with the flow, use a light touch, and trust the process." They also may be viewed as being "wishy-washy" and unable to "stand firm" on their beliefs and decisions.

Water and Secretions

Water is associated with body secretions. Saliva is Ether in Water. Sweat is Air in Water. Urine is Fire in Water, semen or vaginal fluid is Water in Water. Blood and

Lymph is Earth in Water. Disturbances in any of these areas indicate unbalanced proportions of Water to the other elements.

Water and the Body

Water has its positive pole in the breast and lymph areas, ruled by the sign of Cancer. Its neutral pole is in the genitals, ruled by Scorpio, and its negative pole in the feet, ruled by Pisces. "Watery" people are easily able to go with the flow, sometimes resulting in taking a form imposed by someone else. Remembering that water will conform to its container and change shape according to the "temperature." The flow of Water may be interrupted by both internal and external events. In nature, if Water is contained in a pool without access to flow, it becomes stagnant. Air bubbling through Water results in clarity and renewal. The Water element in our bodies interacts with all other elements in profound ways.

Water and Dis-Ease

Problems in the following areas may indicate an imbalance of the Water energies:

- Breast lumps or tenderness
- Herpes
- Menstrual problems
- Prostate problems
- Foot problems
- Pelvic and lower back problems
- Skin problems (in association with the Fire element)
- Oversensitivity to touch
- Allergies

Balancing Water

The Water element is associated with the negative (receiving) energy of the ring finger and fourth toe. A very simple way to encourage the flow of Water is to massage these digits. Try it the next time you are feeling stagnant or confined and let the flow, flow!

Another technique that is useful for balancing the Water element is called the "Five-Pointed Star." Sit or lie down in a comfortable position. Touch your left pelvic area with your right palm, and your right upper chest area with your left palm, fingertips touching left shoulder. Gentle rest both hands in this position until you feel "complete." You may feel a sense of relaxation of muscles, or a tingle of energy, or simply a feeling of satisfaction. Then move your upper hand to rest gently on your throat. This is the contact point for the top of the five-pointed star that you are making on your torso. Again wait for a sense of completion to occur. Now do the same contacts on the opposite hip and shoulder. Touch your right pelvic area with your left palm and your left shoulder area with your right palm. Wait for the relaxation to occur. Then place your right hand gently over your throat. Feel the energy beginning to move and flow. Finally, hug yourself by crossing your arms and placing your hands on opposite shoulders. Relax and feel the flow of the Water element through out your body. Feel Water mixing with Air to stimulate you, mixing with Fire to calm you, and flowing into the space of Ether. Feel the new balance and flow.

Remember the polarity of your hands from chapter 21. Your left hand is a negative (receptive) charge, while your right hand is a positive (giving) charge. You can connect the poles of Water element on your body simply by using your hands. Place one hand on your breast/upper chest area and the other hand on your lower abdominal/pelvic area. Gently massage your lower abdomen and feel the energy begin to open and flow between it and your chest. Now move one hand down to your pelvic area, and bend your leg so that your foot comes into reach of your other hand. Massage your foot and feel the energy flowing between foot and pelvis. To flow energy downward, use your left hand as the "bottom" one, keeping it closer to your feet than your right hand. To flow energy upward, use your left hand at the "top," keeping it closer to your head than your right hand. (Remember, energy flows from positive to negative, from your "positive," or giving, right hand to your "negative," or receiving, left hand.)

Summary

Balanced Water brings a sense of calmness and flow into your life. You are able to flow around obstacles or gently wear them down. You have a new sense of harmony and trust, as your deeper emotions flow towards the surface and become cleansed and renewed. Trust the process of flow in your life today.

Twenty-six

Earth

Earth is dense, passive, and fertile. Earth is the great provider, associated with permanency and stability. Earth provides shelter and protection. Earth provides clay, brick, wood, and food. Associated with the 1st or root chakra, the Earth element provides the grounding necessary to exist on the physical plane. Earth also has the capacity for absorbing other elements in this manifestation process. Earthy people are "down to earth," "grounded," and "solid." Place an Earth person in the room with an Air person and just watch what happens. The airy personality will be standing, pacing, circling around the earthy person, seated comfortably and just observing.

We need the quality of Earth to ground our ideas and manifest our dreams. Earth brings our thoughts down to reality and provides a stable foundation for building our lives.

Earth and Form

Earth is associated with bodily forms. Hair is Ether in Earth, skin is Air in Earth, blood vessels are Fire in Earth, muscles are Water in Earth and bones are Earth in Earth. Disturbances in any of these areas indicate unbalanced proportions of Earth to the other elements. The common concern of osteoporosis with aging indicates a lack of the Earth element. As we grow older, we are more active in our thoughts (Ether/Air) than with our bodies. Physical activities, especially in natural settings, increase the Earth element regardless of age.

Earth and the Body

Earth has its positive pole in the neck area, ruled by the sign of Taurus. Its neutral pole is in the colon, ruled by Virgo, and its negative pole in the knees, ruled by Capricorn. Knees and bowels are common areas of concern with aging. Too much Earth energy slows down the digestive system and clogs the space in the joints. Too little accounts for fragility of hair, skin and bones. Gardening is a great way to increase Earth energy easily. Being out in nature, feeling the earth through your fingertips connects one with earth itself. Stretching, reaching and bending loosen the joints and returns flexibility and space to the body.

Earth and Dis-Ease

Problems in the following areas may indicate an imbalance of the Earth energies:

- Osteoporosis
- Constipation
- Colitis
- Spastic colon
- Hemorrhoids
- Chronic tension in the neck, abdomen, or knees

Balancing Earth

The Earth element is associated with the positive (giving) energy of the little finger and toe. A very simple way to encourage the flow of Earth is to massage these digits. Use it to ground yourself when you are feeling spacey or "out of it."

Earth energy may be balanced easily by a technique known as the Earth Button. Place two fingers of your left hand directly above the pubic bone and two fingers of your right hand just below the lower lip. Massage gently with the two upper fingers and then gently hold both contacts. Breathe deeply, visualizing the movement of energy down the center of your body. Add looking up and down with your eyes (without moving your head) to assist the top-bottom connection. When you feel the energy flow is complete, remove your hands from their contacts. Finish by looking around in a downward direction. Downward eye placement activates the top/bottom dimension of the brain. This emphasizes the feeling of stability and anchors in a feeling of being grounded.

Remember the polarity of your hands from chapter 21. Your left hand is a negative (receptive) charge, while your right hand is a positive (giving) charge. You can connect the poles of Earth element on your body simply by using your hands. Place one hand on your neck and the other hand on your lower abdominal area. Gently massage your lower abdomen and feel the energy begin to open and flow between it and your neck. Now move one hand down to your abdominal area, and place your other hand on your knee. Massage your knee and feel the energy flowing between knee and abdomen. To flow energy downward, use your left hand as the "bottom" one, keeping it closer to your feet than your right hand. To flow energy upward, use your left hand at the "top," keeping it closer to your head than your right hand. (Remember, energy flows from positive to negative, from your "positive," or giving, right hand to your "negative," or receiving, left hand.)

Summary

Balanced Earth brings a sense of grounding into your life. You are able to turn your ideas into reality and see them take form. Time spent in nature; sitting on the ground, playing in the dirt, stimulate the Earth energy. So take a break and go hug a tree. Tell your boss/family/friends that you are just doing your "therapy" to balance your energy. Maybe they will even join you!

Twenty-seven

Polarity Energy Summary and Self-Balancing

The chapters in this section described the five elements that invest the physical body with form and the mind with thought. Ether governs the spaces within the body, and disturbances appear most often as joint problems. Air rules movement within the body and is associated with functioning of the lungs, heart, and nervous system. Fire provides the heat for digestion and body temperature. Water is associated with the genital and reproductive areas of the body, and body liquids. Earth element rules the bones.

The elements travel through the body in biomagnetic waves, going from positive (+) through neutral (0) to negative (-) poles. Air polarizes in the shoulder (+), kidneys (0), calves (-). Fire in the head (+), solar plexus (0) thighs (-). Water includes the breasts (+), pelvis (0), and feet (-). Earth poles are neck (+), bowels (0) knees (-). Polarity works to unblock stuck flows by connecting the energy between each pole. Similar to cleaning a water pipe of leaves, once the flow is cleared, the body's own self-healing functions freely.

Polarity Self-Balancing combines nutrition, visualization, sound, reflexes, and exercise to promote well being. The following are some simple techniques to balance the five elements.

Nutrition

Food increases the flow and potency of elements. Air foods grow high above the ground, including fruits and nuts. Seeds and grains growing above the ground (sesame and sunflower seed, corn, wheat, rice, beans) increase the Fire of digestion. Water foods growing nearest to the ground (green vegetables and melons) balance a fiery system adding a sense of flow to the body. Comfort foods of Earth grow under the ground (potatoes, carrots, onions, beets) and provide a sense of grounding and stability.

When you wish to strengthen an element, eat more of the foods that nourish it. For example, in the heat of summer we tend to eat more Water foods—melons, cantaloupes and so forth—to cool the summer heat and Fire element. In the Winter, to warm up and increase the Fire element, we often consume more grains and breads. We naturally select the foods we need and can consciously reinforce these selections based on Polarity theories.

Visualizations

To increase the flow of an element, simply visualize its properties. Imagine feeling the wind moving to increase Air. Watch a blazing campfire to increase Fire. To cool Fire, imagine floating on the ocean. When feeling "spacey," pretend you are moving down into a cave in the earth. Or actually do them! Stand outside in the wind. Take your shoes off and walk on the earth. Walk in a cool mountain stream. The body responds quickly to real or imagined changes of scenery.

Sounds

Each element is associated with a particular sound. Vowel sounds can balance the elements. Say or sing the following sounds aloud, repeating each three times. Sing "Aaaaa" to expand Ether in the throat. Feel Air moving in the chest while singing "Eeeee." Feel "Iiiiii," the sound of Fire, in the solar plexus, Water, "Ooooo," in the pelvic area, and "Uuuuu," Earth, deep at the base of the spine. When feeling out of balance, repeat the sound that soothes your mind/body state. Water and Earth calm Air and Fire. Use O or U when under stressful activity to calm down. When feeling low and lethargic, energize yourself by singing E or I.

Polarity Reflexes

The energy of the elements run through our fingers and toes. By holding and massaging a particular finger or toe, we can balance individual currents and flows within the entire body. Ether is the neutral thumb and big toe. Air is the negatively charged index finger and second toe. Fire is the positively charged middle finger and third toe. Water is the negatively charged ring finger and fourth toe. Earth is the positively charged little finger and toe. Reflect on the common use of the Fire finger for anger and the ring finger for love and you will see their connection with the elements.

Polarity Exercises

A few basic exercises, done daily for two-three minutes without stress or strain can balance the elements. Check with your medical advisor prior to beginning any new exercise program.

The squat is used to bring all elements into balance. Bend your knees and squat down, with elbows at knees and hands holding the bottom of your feet. Gently rock while in this position. When performing this exercise, try to have your feet flat on the floor, and your knees behind your toes. You may place a book under your heels at first to maintain this position without undue stress.

The cliffhanger balances Ether and Air. Stand, place the heels of your hands on a firm table behind you, and slide your bottom straight down, bending your knees and keeping your elbows close together. Feel the stretch between your shoulder blades as the muscles gently lengthen and relax. Do not strain. Repeat two or three times.

Punching balances Fire. Stand, both hands in a fist, take a breath and push your right hand out forcibly while shouting "HA!" Breathe in while punching left hand out. Shout loudly! Really release the pent-up Fire that has been repressed inside.

The scissor kick balances Water. Lie on your stomach, bend your knees, and swing your lower legs back and forth across each other. Feel the muscles in your hips and pelvis begin to relax. Make the movements gentle and smooth. Just kick and relax!

The cerebral spinal bounce balances Earth. Stand, feet apart, hands on thighs, arms straight. Bend knees and gently "bounce" body in rhythmical movement. You may rock back and forth or from side to side. Gently feel the flow of energy going downward, grounding through your feet into the earth below.

Most of all, listen to your own body and do the exercises within your comfort zone.

Energy Precedes Form

All dis-ease is a byproduct of an imbalanced energy system. Our energy becomes disorganized when we experience mental, emotional, or physical strain or trauma. Energy can easily be realigned. Once the blocks are removed, we can connect fully with the eternal Source of Energy, Balance and Health. Table 6 at right provides a summary of Polarity Self-Balancing.

Listen to your body and feel the flow of energy. Notice times when you feel stiff and stagnant and bring in Air and Fire. Notice the times when you feel hyper and spacey and bring in Earth and Water. May you always be in the flow of your life.

	Ether	Air	Fire	Water	Earth
Summary	*Emotions*	*Movement*	*Metabolism*	*Secretions*	*Body Forms*
Sense	Hearing	Touch	Sight	Taste	Smell
Function	Expression, space	Movement, diversity, expansion	Motivation, will, drive, upward flow	Creativity, sexuality, downward flow	Structure, crystallization
Body System	Joints	Respiratory, nervous, circulatory	Metabolism, digestion	Reproductive, lymphatic, body fluids	Waste, elimination, skeletal
Emotions	+ return to spirit; - grief	+ compassion, charity, love; - desire, judgment	+ forgiveness, enthusiasm; - anger, resentment	+ letting go; - attachment	+ courage; - fear
Polarity Points	Above to below each joint	Shoulders to mid-back to calves	Forehead to solar plexus to thighs	Breast area to pelvis to feet	Neck to bowels to knees
Polarity Reflexology Qualities	0 Big toe 0 Thumb	- Second toe - Index finger	+ Third toe + Middle finger	- Fourth toe - Ring finger	+ Little toe + Little finger
	Head is positive (+), trunk is neutral (0), feet are negative (-). The left hand is negative (receiving) and the right hand is positive (giving).				
Foods		Foods highest above the ground: fruits and nuts, citrus fruits, nuts	Foods grown higher above the ground: seeds and grains: sesame, sunflower, corn, wheat, rice	Foods grown above and nearest ground: vegetables, cucumbers, melons, tomatoes, strawberries, seafood	Foods grown underground and near the surface: potatoes, carrots, beets, onions, garlic, herb roots
Visualizations	Imagine an openness in your throat and the ability to express yourself freely.	Feel the breath as it flows in and out of your nose.	Imagine watching a blazing campfire and feel its warmth	Imagine floating on the ocean, feeling the waves rise and fall.	Imagine sitting in a deep, earthy forest. Think slowly and take your time.
Sound	Repeat the vowel sound "A"	Repeat the vowel sound "E"	Repeat the vowel sound "I"	Repeat the vowel sound "O"	Repeat the vowel sound "U"
Sight	Look at the color blue	Look at the color green	Look at the color yellow	Look at the color orange	Look at the color red

Table 6. Polarity Energy Element Summary and Activities

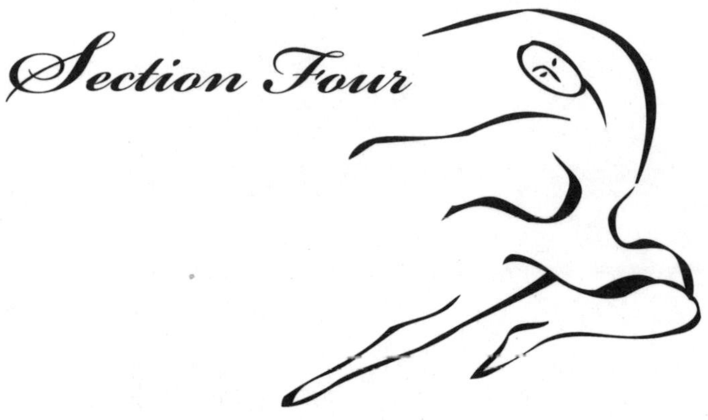

Section Four

Feng Shui: The Energy of Your Environment

Feng Shui (pronounced "fung shway") is the idea of living in harmony and balance with our environment and dates back over seven-thousand years. It is the study of energy (Chi) and how its circulation affects people. The circulation of this invisible energy can be blocked or distorted by our environment, thus creating Shar Chi (or negative energy).

There are many different schools of Feng Shui in China. For example, the Form School, which began in southern China with its varied landscape, studies the natural environment-mountains, lakes, streams and seeks to place buildings and dwellings in harmony with the landscape. The Compass School originated in northern China's relatively flat landscape and relies on the cardinal directions for proper arrangement of a room, office, or home.

This section describes practical applications of the Compass School in the placement of colors, symbols, and other auspicious objects according the compass directions. In addition, we will explore the belief systems that govern our internal environment and discover how they affect and effect the external environment.

Twenty-eight

Basic Principles of Feng Shui

Feng Shui is about being in harmony with nature and your environment. Many things we do, such as cleaning a room of clutter when we feel depressed, are actually Feng Shui tools. The idea of being in balance is hard for the Western mind to grasp.

The Balance of Yin and Yang

This concept of opposites in perfect balance is called Yin and Yang in the East. Yin and Yang are opposites that are constantly evolving and cycling. In this balance are transformation, interaction, and interdependence. Look at the symbol of Yin and Yang for a moment.

Within the dark (yin) is the light of yang. Within the light of yang is the dark of yin. Even the words dark and light have different meaning in terms of Feng Shui. Yin is the dark, the night, the negative (receiving) force of energy associated with the moon, water, and feminine qualities. Yang is sunny, light, positive (sending) force of energy associated with fire, the summer, and masculine qualities. It is for natural winter to follow summer, for the day to follow the night. They give each other meaning and need each other to exist.

According to Feng Shui, the dance of opposites of yin and yang maintain the balance of the cosmos. We, too, in our environments, require a balance of opposites. Imagine living in an all white room, with the lights on all the time. In this room the floor is white, all the furniture is white and the light never ends. How long could you stay in such a room? An hour, a day, a week? With nothing to contrast, with nothing to stand out, what would your life be like? Now into this room add some yin. Turn off the lights at night. Add a black sofa and a black coffee table. The room improves because there is more contrast, and therefore more balance. Now add variations of color between white and black. A green rug. Blue walls. Yellow flowers. Now the room becomes livable. Now you can feel at home.

Feng Shui uses colors and textures and objects all designed to create a balance and harmony in any environment. When you bring your environment into harmony, you are able to flow your energies better. You are able to accomplish more with less stress. And you attract to you balance and harmony in affairs of your life.

Feng Shui Cures

Feng Shui Cures or Remedies are objects in the environment that can shift energy when necessary to attain balance. In Feng Shui, negative energy is called "Shar Chi." Negative energy occurs when there are physical or emotional blocks to the flow of energy. For example: Before we moved to the mountains, my husband and I lived in a hundred year old Southern farmhouse with windows everywhere and doors opening off of every room (to catch the breeze on a hot summer day). There were very little blocks to energy flow in that old house. Our new house in the mountains lacked that old Southern flowing design. The rooms felt small and closed, with fewer windows and doors. We immediately went out and bought mirrors for each room. The mirrors opened up the space and reflected the beautiful mountains inside. Without realizing it, we were using a Feng Shui Cure. We hadn't even heard of the term Feng Shui at that time, we just knew that we needed to open up the space.

You have probably used Cures without knowing why. Most cures are a combination of common sense and good taste. There are 8 basic cures in Feng Shui. These cures are used to generate energy when the structure of the room or building prevents an open energy flow. Feng Shui Cures include the use of:

- *Bright objects:* Mirrors, faceted crystal balls, gems, lights, candles, etc.
- *Sounds:* Wind chimes, bells, music
- *Living chi:* Flowers, plants, birds, fish
- *Moving objects:* mobiles, chimes, fountains
- *Heavy objects:* Stone sculptures, furniture
- *Mechanical items:* Computers, stereos, TVs
- *Bamboo items:* Flutes, etc.
- *Color:* Relates to each area on Baqua Map

There are also belief cures for our internal environment. In each of the following chapters we will discuss both external and internal cures for living in balance and harmony.

The Baqua (or Ba'Gua)

In arranging an environment, nine areas are noted to be of special significance. These nine areas also reflect the major aspects of life.

The Baqua Map in Table 8 shows the nine separate areas of energy and intention in Feng Shui. Baqua means eight-sided and is pictured as an octagonal shape. You may superimpose the map over any floor plan of a home, room, or office to see what areas need attention. Chapters in this section review the nine areas of the Baqua with respect to both the external environment and how it reflects our inner beliefs.

Feng Shui and Beliefs

Feng Shui literally means "wind and water." Wind is the unseen, while water is the visible, the manifest. The universe is composed of these two forces of energy or nature. What we believe (wind) is reflected in our environment (water). And what we see in our environment reflects our beliefs.

A belief is a combination of thought and feeling that is buried deep in the subconscious mind. Subconscious beliefs hold energy, Chi, and express this energy in both subtle and powerful ways. The "collective unconsciousness," a term coined by psychologist Carl Jung, is a pool of cultural beliefs that have an influence on society and the individual. One of the benefits of viewing Feng Shui through the Baqua Map is an opportunity to categorize our beliefs and view them through the reflection of our environment. Then we can use the environment to reinforce a positive belief, or change a negative one.

The chapters in this section review each of the nine aspects of life according to Feng Shui principles and our cultural beliefs in relation to these nine aspects of life. Each chapter contains practical information about changing our environment and our beliefs to add more Chi and balance.

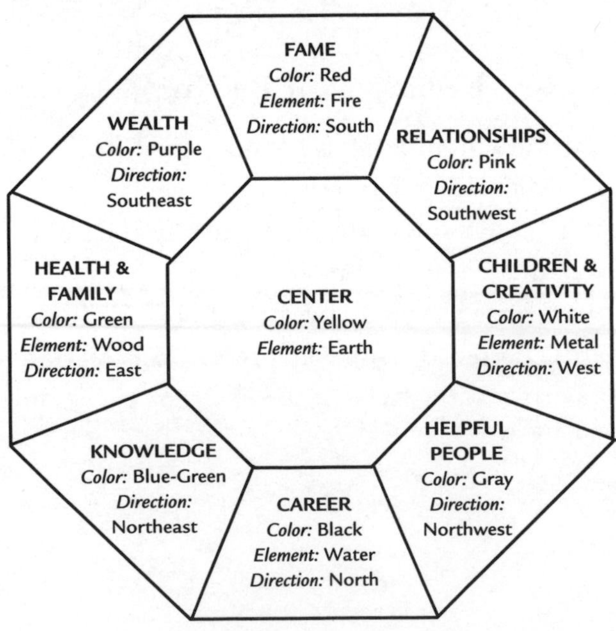

TABLE 7. THE BAQUA MAP

Twenty-nine

The East: Health & Family

The East represents the area in your home or office that holds the energy of home, health, and family. This area is associated with active participation, new ideas and reaching out, as well as physical and emotional healing and support.

Environment

Wood is the element associated with the East in Feng Shui. It represents spring, the beginning of the cycle of life. Wood contains growth, creation and nourishment. Objects that reinforce this element in your environment include: tall cylinders, rectangles, green floral patterns, plants and flowers. Some schools of Feng Shui say that wood in your home or office must be living, such as small shrubs or bonsai trees. Others say that it is okay to include wood floors and furniture as an aspect of this element. The debate is whether "dead wood" counts or if wood must be living to contain balancing Chi.

The color green is associated with the East and healing, prosperity, luck, fertility and harmony. It is probably no coincidence that operating room scrubs are green. I wonder if the physicians know they are using Feng Shui in the operating room?

Take a moment to look at the East area of your home, room or office. Does it contain any Wood elements? Is there anything green? Are there any blocks to the flow of energy such as clutter? For now, just make a mental note and read on!

Beliefs

What are your beliefs about health and healing? Traditional medicine holds the belief that the body is mechanical in nature and that the mind is separate from the body. To fix the mind, alter the chemicals in the body. To fix the body, remove the diseased part or suppress the symptoms with medicine. Energy medicine, based upon the work of Einstein, believes that the body consists of energy suspended in a timeless, flowing field. Modern physicists have shown that matter is actually composed of quanta, which in turn are made of invisible vibrations. These invisible vibrations can actually be measured as the electromagnetic waves the each person emits.

If you believe that the body is a machine and the mind has no influence upon the machine, then your health becomes a matter of accepting the fortunes of fate and genetics as you watch your body become old and diseased. However, if you believe that your body is pure energy and that the combination of your thoughts, feelings and beliefs can influence that energy, then you have a powerful tool for health and healing.

There is a balance between these two opposites. If you break a leg, it is probably easier to have a mechanical solution, a cast, than to try to heal the break with the energy of your mind alone. However, if you have been diagnosed with a disease (a complex of related signs and symptoms), perhaps you can change your belief enough to consider it a dis-ease or a lack of ease in the energy flow in your body. This opens you up to exploring the energies of beliefs and emotions as a part of your healing.

What beliefs do you currently hold about your own body? Do you believe the commercials that announce, "it's cold and flu season" and get a cold every winter? Do believe that because a relative had cancer, that you will have it too? Do you believe that it is natural to have more aches and pains as you grow older? Begin to clear out the self-prophecy of old beliefs, just as you clear out the clutter of your home or office. I am not telling you to ignore your body or forgo preventative medical check-ups. I am asking you to look at what you are reinforcing in your body. Your body responds to your commands, especially when there is a firm belief behind them. (Remember, the definition of belief is thought combined with emotion) Why not tell your body something different? Myrtle Fillmore, co-founder the Unity Church, described in one of her articles what she called her "discovery." Myrtle was diagnosed with tuberculosis in the 1880s, when there was no medical cure. She began talking to the cells in her body. She talked to her lungs and told them to heal. She talked to every cell and atom in her body, loved them, sent good wishes to them, and she healed completely. The body responded to her mental energy and beliefs that she could heal.

In another healing story, a woman was diagnosed with cancer and told that she had only three months to live. Because she did not have anything to lose, she called her friend who was living in the Caribbean and asked her to make an appointment for her with a local "witch doctor." She arrived at the doctor's office and he examined her, and then said: "Man in white coat put curse on you. I remove the curse." With that, the "curse" was removed, and the woman healed completely! What healed her if not a change in belief that resulted in a change in her own energy vibrations that healed the cancer? The world is full of wonderful miracles of energy when we believe. That was one of the strong messages from the New Testament—believe and it will be true for you. Belief works because we are energy beings at our core.

Cures

Feng Shui Cures to increase health, healing, and family harmony involve the use of Wood elements, the color green, auspicious symbols, and the belief that what you are doing is going to work!

When using cures in this area, affirm you positive intention to heal yourself or your family. Believe that the universe is energy, and that thoughts, feeling, and objects can affect energy. Affirm that energy is now flowing freely in your body, your mind, and your environment. Affirm the power of energy to heal and relieve any condition that is currently distressing you. Focus your attention on the healing that is now occurring and the well being that is coming into your life.

Clear out clutter in your mind as you first clear out clutter in the East area of your room or office. Look at the area and notice, which things give you a sense of health, vitality and healing and which do not. For example, if the east area of your home is the mudroom, and there is always dirty footwear, discarded towels, and other messes—notice how that makes you feel. Begin to re-arrange the area to gain a sense of cleanliness, orderliness, and harmony. Bring in the Wood element of this area by adding a living plant. Lucky bamboo *(Dracaena Sanderana)* is a small bamboo plant that lives in indirect sunlight and at extreme temperature ranges and only needs water to grow in (no soil). It is a perfect plant for the health area of a room or office because bamboo is wood, yet it is green!

Another great place to use live wood is when your staircase empties into your doorway. This is considered negative Chi in Feng Shui. The cure is to place a live, potted shrub at the bottom of the staircase. This enlivens the area and creates good Chi.

In Chinese folklore, the Dragon is associated with the East and the spirit of change and transformation, while the turtle is associated with longevity, strength, and endurance. Placing a small statue of a dragon or a turtle in the East area of your room will add the Chi of long family life and harmony. There is even an object called a Treasure Turtle Dragon that is often used in this area. This statue shows a turtle riding on the back of a dragon whose body is a turtle shell. Combined, the statue represents strength, goodness, longevity for the family and the individual.

Put personal objects that reaffirm your intention for good health and family harmony in the East. Place a photo of your family on vacation, relaxing, enjoying each other in perfect health. Write our healing affirmations and pin them up. Make a colleague of the most healing pictures and words you can find, frame it, and place it in the East. Be careful not to crowd the area. One or two objects that represent health and family will do nicely. Above all, keep the area neat, clean, and healthy looking and feeling!

Thirty

The Southeast: Wealth

The Southeast is the area in your environment that represents wealth. It is associated with good fortune and moneymaking. Wealth is a symbol of abundant energy flow and the freedom to do what needs to be done in the service of self and others.

Environment

There is no single Feng Shui element associated with this area. In the translation between elements in the Creative cycle, the Wood of the east moves southeast to nourish the Fire of the south. Combining these elements, one may say that the Wood makes Fire and promotes higher purpose, laughter, meeting new people and embracing life.

The color associated with this area is purple, the color of nobility and royalty. The energy of the color purple includes aspects of spirituality, wisdom, honor and psychic awareness. Perhaps one must have psychic awareness to acquire wealth in today's society!

Look at the southeast portion of your home, room, or office. Does anything in it remind you of wealth at this time? Is there any room to receive wealth? Any open spaces? Any signs of flow and movement? Is there any hint of purple or its tones of violet and indigo? Analyze this area for anything that feels to you like it is blocking wealth and for anything that seems to be attracting wealth. I know this sounds subjective, but energy, like the wind, is very subjective. We cannot see the air, but we can feel it as a breeze gently caresses our cheeks. We cannot see the energy of wealth, but we know the instant we feel rich—just as we know the instant that we feel poor.

Beliefs

Do you believe in the Law of Scarcity or the Law of Abundance? The Law of Scarcity holds that we live in a limited universe, on a limited planet, and in a limited life based on the sheer good will of others or on the fortunes of fate. At any time what we have may be taken from us, depending entirely upon the greed of others. The stock market falls, our boss fires us using the politically correct term of downsizing, our funds dry up. And there is no more because there is only a limited amount for everyone, and we seem to have used up our share.

The Law of Abundance holds that we live in an infinite universe, on a planet that is self-renewing and has enough arable land to feed all its inhabitants, and in a limitless life full of possibility and adventure. Our fortunes depend upon our abilities to let go of anxiety and worry and embrace the all-providing spirit of plenty.

The spirit of wealth and plenty is manifested as money and money is a form of exchange. In itself it means nothing. What it represents means everything. What does money mean to you? Does it mean freedom to go where you wish and do what you want? Does it mean security to provide a roof over your head and food to eat? Does it mean feeling important and successful? Whatever it means to you is at the core of your beliefs about money. This belief core is buried very deep inside each one of us. The saying "The rich get richer and the poor get poorer" is a statement about beliefs. When you feel rich, money comes to you freely. When you feel poor, each dollar is a struggle to obtain and retain. So the secret to wealth is to feel wealthy deep inside, to change your belief to feel that you are good enough to be wealthy or that you do deserve to be wealthy.

I truly wish I could say that changing beliefs about money is easy. Perhaps by the time this book is published I will be saying that. Right now though, I am in the transition process of changing beliefs. I am in the process of releasing a core belief that I can make all the money I wish *as long as I am working on salary for someone else.* Through the first twenty-five years of my professional life as a physical therapist, I worked for someone else—mostly at large institutions such as hospitals and academic universities. Money was easy to make. All I had to do was show up each day and I received my paycheck. I loved what I was doing and loved helping people become stronger, recover from accident or illness, and be relieved of pain. That is a part of making money also, loving what you do. Ten years ago I left my salaried position to open my own business. The business was successful in that it paid for itself and its expenses, but I could never find enough money to pay myself. After several years, I returned to a salaried position in physical therapy. I retreated into the area where I knew (believed) that I could make money. And I did. I paid off all my debts and once again enjoyed patient care. But some higher voice kept calling to me. There was something else I was meant to do. There was a lesson to be learned about money that I could never learn while working for someone else. So, seven years ago I went into partnership with my husband and we opened our own business.

Now owning your own business is a unique way to learn about money. Money does not come into a business just because you show up for work each day. In fact, some days, such as today as I am writing this, money does not come in at all. I can't *will* customers and clients to enter my door. In fact, when I want money most, I have the fewest customers. Like when bills come in and I become worried about paying them. What, you may be asking, does this have to do with belief systems? Owning your own business is a great way to monitor how you are feeling deep inside. On the days I feel wealthy, customers and clients pour through the door and bombard the website. It doesn't matter if it is snowing and sleeting outside or 110 degrees. They find their way to us and give us money for our products and services. However, on the days I am feeling poor, I interact with no one. The phone doesn't ring, the website has no visitors, and I can spend eight hours without talking with another human being. There is a great book I have mentioned before called *Excuse Me, Your Life is Waiting* by Lynn Grabhorn that explores this issue of feelings in relation to money. I highly recommend reading it if you are considering allowing money to be a life lesson you are ready to learn.

Belief in wealth, being able to attain wealth, is vital to having money. As we explore each of the nine areas of the Baqua, you will find at least one area that seems to be a core belief that is currently creating great obstacles for you. Money is my issue. Yours may be health or relationships or creativity. I believe that when we place ourselves in the position to confront our core lesson(s), we have firmly stepped onto the spiritual path. The path to wealth can be very spiritual. Lasting wealth and abundance requires faith and trust and openness. It requires that ability to hold money loosely, to risk fortunes because you know that eventually you will gain them back and even more. The road to riches is paved with many who try and try again, convinced that this time things will work out. The successful turn their talents over to God, a Higher Source, instinct, whatever term they may use and allow themselves to be guided into wealth. Check back with me in a few years and I'll tell you where I am on this wonderful (and sometimes scary) path. For now, let's return to Feng Shui and ways to bring wealth into your environment.

Cures

Feng Shui has many cures for Wealth. Again, use a cure with the intention to help you change your belief about your relationship to Wealth. Let each change you make in your Wealth area reflect new beliefs about abundance and Wealth coming to you easily and quickly.

Feng Shui cures involve attracting Wealth to you rather than getting Wealth by effort and activity. They are symbols that remind you to allow Wealth and abundance to flow easily into your life.

For good fortune and money making, place a Prosperity Frog (Three-Legged Toad) in your Wealth area. The origins of this belief date back to tenth century China, when the Minister of State Lui Hai was said to have possessed a three-legged toad that would convey him to any place he wished to go. To retain the toad, he would bait a line with gold coins and the toad would always return to him. Today the toad (or frog) represents auspicious symbols of abundance and prosperity.

Ever wonder why Chinese restaurants have fish aquariums and statues of Buddhas and cats by the cash register? The fish is included as one of the auspicious signs on the footprints of the Buddha and signifies freedom of restraints or obstructions. Live fish, swimming in aquariums, represent the flow of wealth and money and career success. Figures of Buddha Laughing remind us to keep our sense of humor even in times of financial trouble. Buddha is often represented as traveling across the county with a sack on his back or sitting in a Ru-Yi bowl of plenty, always spreading joy, prosperity and happiness. Lucky Cats, holding the Chinese symbols for good fortune and wealth, are often placed near a cash register. In China, the cat is a natural protector of silkworms and therefore a source of financial success in business. Lucky Cats are said to bring prosperity to any home or business.

Additional Feng Shui cures to attract money include the use of Lucky Red Envelopes and ancient Chinese coins. Originally Chinese coins were used as amulets of protection against negative energy. They became symbols of energy as they were used for money, just like money is used today. According to legend, placing three or five Chinese coins in a red envelope and then placing the envelope in your Wealth area will attract money to you. Adding a personal affirmation of your willingness to receive money will enhance the energy. It is certainly worth a try, don't you think?

Finally, view the Wealth area of your home or business with an eye for the things that represent wealth to you. What objects make you feel wealthy by just looking at them? They need not be expensive objects, but they must generate the energy of wealth and money. My favorite aunt and uncle were wealthy, or at least wealthy to me. They lived in a wonderful home with lots of rooms to explore on wooded acres of land. I received one item after their death, a brass stamp holder sitting on top of a marble base. That stamp holder was always on my uncle's desk in his home office. It represents wealth to me because it was his and he used it to grow a successful business. I recently found the stamp holder in a box that I hadn't unpacked for years and years. The holder is now firmly in place in the Wealth area of my business. Each time I look at it, I feel wealthy. Find an object the helps you feel wealthy and view it often!

Another energy technique is to pile money on top of a mirror. Use loose change and paper bills. Allow the reflection in the mirror to multiply your money. As with all areas, be sure your Wealth area is free of clutter, neat, and clean. Allow some emptiness so that there is space to receive money. Relax and enjoy money flowing into your life.

Thirty-one

The South: Fame & Success

The South represents the area in your home or office that holds the energy of fame and success. This area is associated with enthusiasm, courage, vitality, and good fortune.

Environment

Fire is the element associated with the South in Feng Shui. Fire represents life energy and action. It is the summer, the peak of the natural cycle. Objects that reinforce this element include triangular, pointed and angular shapes, and red designs in fabrics and carpets and artwork. The use of candles, incense, and sage smudge also introduce the element of fire into the environment.

The color red is associated with your Fame and Success area. Red represents love, passion, energy, and attracts recognition, respect, confidence and luck. Red aids in motivation and inspiration, open-heartedness, fun, laughter and networking. Variations of the color red are also appropriate for this area including purple (the heart of fire), and orange.

Look now at the South portion of your room, home, or business. Does it contain any of the elements of fire? Are there any candles or the color red anywhere? Does this area of your dwelling look successful? What reminds you of success when you look South? Hold these thoughts as we move on to beliefs.

Beliefs

What are your beliefs about fame and success? The classic paradigm here is pessimism vs. optimism. A pessimistic person is one who looks on the worst side of everything and who has the tendency to exaggerate in thought the evils of life. An optimistic person believes that things are all right and takes a cheerful and hopeful view of life. The optimist believes in the doctrine that all is for the best and has the habit of looking at the brighter side of life.

Now, you are probably thinking that you know many people who are successful pessimists. People who appear negative and yet are highly successful. But appearances can be deceiving. The truly successful person is an optimist deep down inside. He or she believes that they can and will succeed—and they do. The successful person is also a consistent person. During a Winter Olympics several years ago, one of the gold medal winners was interviewed about his success. When asked how he felt about winning, he said, "I felt good yesterday, I feel good today, and I will feel good tomorrow." That is an attitude of success!

In what areas of your life are you currently a success? Perhaps you are a successful parent, or artist, or businessperson. In what areas do you wish to become more successful? Look at these two areas side by side. What are the differences in your feelings between these two areas? Can you pinpoint the feeling that motivates each area—the area of success and the area of nonsuccess? Feelings that motivate success come from beliefs that you can and will be able to do something or have something. Feelings that motivate failure come from feelings of lack and unworthiness, the underlying feeling of fear.

Try this simple exercise. Think about an area in which you wish to be more successful. Close your eyes and connect with the feelings you have when you picture success in the area. Now think about an area in your life in which you are now, or have been in the past, very successful. Close your eyes again and think about the feelings you experience when you remember your success. Very gently, with eyes closed, transfer those successful feelings from the past to the success you desire in the future. Begin to feel the success coming to you. You will have completed the exercise when you hold the same feelings about your future success as you have about your past success. Every time you think about the areas of success you desire, note your feelings—and bring forward into the present those joyous, awesome feelings of success from the past. By your consistent feelings of joy and confidence, success will come to you.

Cures

First, clear all the clutter from the South/Success area of your home, room or business. Organize an area for work in this space. You may have a small table or simply a notepad where you can write down your ideas and plans for success. In Feng Shui, the work area is to be organized so you always face the door. It is believed that when your back is to the door you are vulnerable and are inviting competition into your life.

You may also want to take a look at your front door—even if it is not in the South. Is the front of your business or home welcoming success, or are there barriers present? Clutter is one barrier. Dark or closed in feelings around the door are another. Are the porch or steps leading to the door neat and clean, or is there uneven or broken places? Clearing, repairing, adding lights and mirrors all beacon success.

Returning to the South portion of the room, try adding a red candle or a red rose (silk roses are fine!), some incense, or other items that connect with the Fire element. Make a collage of photos that remind you of success. Add personal treasures that bode success for you, remembering not to clutter the area. Have the intention of success each time you view this area. Feel the feeling of success each time you think about this area. Give your self permission to be successful, no matter what anyone else says to you or even thinks about you. Know you are successful and it will come.

Thirty-two

The Southwest: Relationships

The Southwest holds the energy of relationships, marriage, and business partnerships. It is associated with support, sharing, and selflessness.

Environment

No single Feng Shui element is associated with this area. It is the transition between the red of Fire element and the white of the Metal element. The perfect blending of red and white produce pink. Pink is the color of emotional healing, protection, love, support and letting go. In terms of energy, the white light from heaven merges with the red light of earth, blending, soothing, and harmonizing. Pink is often associated with the heart and loving.

Look at the Southwest area of your home or office. What is there that reminds you of love? Again, look for clutter, dust, disorganization. Is your love "dusty"? If you are single, is there any space in this area to invite others into your life? If you are married or living with a partner, is there space for your relationship to unfold? Just note the changes you may wish to make in this area for now.

Beliefs

The basic belief paradigm in this area is the experience of conditional vs. unconditional love. Conditional love in relationships requires that when you do something for someone else, they reciprocate and do something for you. You love the person only if you have visible evidence of their returning love. You love them only when they follow certain unspoken rules you have about behaviors in a relationship. Many of us grew up with one or more parents whose love appeared conditional most of the time. Those of us who were accommodators simply learned the rules and obeyed them. Those who were more rebellious did not follow the rules and often felt rejected.

My brother and I were perfect examples. I know that our mother loved us very deeply, but was brought up in a family that did not show affection. My brother rebelled from day one and simply went his own way. I, however, learned to please my mother at all costs, to anticipate her wishes before she spoke them, and to do what she wanted me to do. It was a total nonverbal relationship. I came to feel that my mother would only love me when I washed the dishes, cleaned my room, walked the dog, smiled all the time, did not pout, and so on. I followed what I believed were the conditions for her love. I was rigid in following those rules, even later in life when I married and was establishing a new relationship with my husband.

One year, when I was thirty-eight years old, on a visit to my parents, I had a sudden epiphany. I had just finished my dissertation and had been awarded my doctoral degree from the University of Georgia. I was rather proud of this accomplishment but my mother said nothing during dinner. After dinner, I sprang up as usual to clear the table and wash the dishes. Mother came out into the kitchen and expressed her disapproval of the way in which I was washing the dishes. Here I was, a Doctor of Education, and I didn't know how to wash dishes! I was crushed. I cried. And I realized how many years I had spent trying to earn my mother's conditional love. That was enough. I decided that there must be a better way. So, I began to watch my father. I had always felt unconditional love from him. He loved and supported me always, even when he admitted that he did not understand why I was doing something that he would not do. I watched him with my mother. And you know what? He loved her unconditionally too! He never judged, criticized, or made her feel unloved in any way. I knew that he had some problems with the way she behaved at times, but his love was always at the forefront.

Unconditional love—what a revelation. It is about never withholding love because of circumstances, values, judgments, or beliefs. You may not like or appreciate what someone else is doing, but you can still have compassion for them, and give your love to them.

In the movie *Kundun*, the authorized story of the life of the Dalai Lama, one scene early in the movie illustrates this type of love. The Dalai Lama is three or four-years old and has just been discovered by the monks who were searching for him. He is held in the arms of a monk, enfolded in his robes. As he looks up at the monk as he is told something like this: "You were born to love. That is your only function. That is why you are here. To love and to have compassion for all beings. You are born to love. That is all." What if every child born were held in loving arms and told that they were born to love and to be loving. What if every child knew they were loved because they exist? No other reason. They were loved and loving. That is all. What kind of a world would we witness if unconditional love were the dominant emotion?

One footnote before we move on. Unconditional love does not mean allowing murder and crime and horrors go on without notice. It does not mean jumping into bed with everyone, or orgies, or flower children throwbacks. Unconditional love reaches past actions, which must be dealt with by society, to the core of love in every one of us. When that core is touched, miracles occur. Hate and violence breed from fear and lack of love. Unconditional love is applying the love we give our pets (and are given back by our pets) to the people we live with, work with, and have interactions with daily. Unconditional love will transform relationship into effortless mutual benefit. That is the powerful Chi in unconditional love.

Cures

The first cure for relationships is to love yourself unconditionally. If you place conditions on your own self-love, then you will place conditions on the love you give to others. If you only love yourself when you accomplish something, when you are healthy, when you do good, then you must, by default, apply that criteria to those around you. Practice loving yourself when you feel bad, when you have just made a mistake, when you have been unkind. Practice loving yourself because you exist, because you are living, because you are here. Meditation will assist you in developing the feelings of unconditional love. The more you understand the transitory nature of reality, the more you will come to know that just being here is enough. Just loving is enough. And when you are full of love inside, you naturally overflow that love into your relationships and to the world. So give yourself permission to love yourself. And then expand that permission to loving others. To be in relationship with others unconditionally will bring good Chi into your life.

On the more tangible side, Feng Shui includes cures to enhance these feelings of love and relationship. In the Southwest area of your room or business, place pairs of things to remind you that you are in relationship. Find two matching candles, pink in color, and set them together. Two Austrian crystals hanging side by side, equally matched, will bring relationship Chi into your area. Two matching mirrors, two matching cushions, two of anything peaceful and loving will do nicely.

Fish tanks or carvings of fish are often placed in this area. In China, the carp fish represents harmony and marital bliss, especially when two of them are seen swimming together against the current. Facing obstacles together has become an emblem of perseverance. The fish symbol may be used in a business or office to enhance relationships between employees and customers.

Since we are on the relationships area, we need to discuss the arrangement of your bedroom—even if it is not in the Southwest of your home. For successful relationships, place the head of the bed against a wall and centered, so that both people can get in without a struggle. The ideal location is to place the bed so you have a clear view of the door from the bed, but not directly in front of a door. In the bedroom, use pairs of things to enhance relationships. Matching night tables on both sides of the bed, matching lights, matching pillows all enhance the energy of relationships.

Finally, in the bedroom, feel free to say—and mean—"I love you" the last thing at night and the first thing in the morning. " Good night, I love you!" and "Good morning, I love you."

Thirty-three

The West: Creativity & Children

The West represents children and creativity. It is associated with intuition, organization, and completing things. We complete our children and then we let them go. We complete our projects and then move on to something else, and we listen to our inner voice of intuition to know when to apply our talents to the next cycle.

Environment

The West is associated with the season of autumn, the waning of the natural cycle, the middle years of life, a time of finishing things by the development of self-discipline accompanied by creative ways to handle life. The element Metal is used in the West to bring the energy of completion and success. Metal frames, brass doorknobs, sculptures, domes, cylinders, and round shapes. Metal is the most common remedy for negative earth energies. The use of copper, silver, gold, and bronze balance and bring harmony. Use of the colors white, silver, gold, and metallic is included in the West. The color white is a blank canvas on which to paint your picture of creativity and fruition. Fun objects, childlike objects, games, and toys are all appropriate for the West. In our store we have filled the Children and Creativity section with fairies, smoky mountain trolls, wizards, coloring books, fiber optic lights, and all things that remind us to enjoy, be in awe, and have fun.

Look at the West of your room or home and seek out the fun. What is creative there? What makes you smile? What reminds you to be young and adventurous? Children live in the now, moment to moment. They draw tremendous creativity from their minds and imaginations. The energy of this area invites you to explore your own creativity and to have fun.

Beliefs

Fear prevents creativity. Joy promotes creativity. That's the paradigm we work with in this area of the Baqua. Fear of failure, fear of being laughed at, fear of not being good enough, all contribute to lack of creativity. Joy in expression, joy in doing for the sake of doing, joy in living all unleash creativity. What do you feel creative at? Perhaps it is cooking, or gardening, or crossword puzzles. How do you feel when you are being creative? You probably feel light, swift, focused, happy, in the zone. These words describe a deeper sense of confidence in knowing what to do or at least how to figure out what to do. Creativity comes in many forms and styles. Everyone is creative.

Belief in your own abilities fosters creativity. Fear of judgment from others limits creativity. I recently saw a TV show in which elephants were painting pictures for sale to provide money for their care. The elephants took the paintbrushes with their trunks, made deliberate strokes on the canvas, and requested different brushes and colors from their owners. One art critic commented that it was not necessarily creative that the elephants could paint. What was creative was that they knew when to stop! The elephants were surely not afraid of judgment or criticism!

To develop creativity is simple. Try something that you have always wanted to do and do it. Treat each "mistake" as a lesson you are learning and begin and begin again. That's the fun, that's the creative part. Do something new and, at first, be satisfied just in the doing. You may uncover a computer nerd, or an artist, or a chef hiding deep inside. Don't give up or listen to the judging voice. Just do it. You will be amazed at the results and at the fun you have had in the process.

Cures

To bring the energy of creativity and creation into your home or office, hang a crystal in a window. The most common hanging crystals are made of leaded glass. The microscopic particles of lead catch the rays of the sun, reflecting them into rainbows across the room. Austrian crystals do nicely and come in a variety of shapes. Crystals draw yang (active) energy into your environment and promote the energy for completion of projects. The miracle of watching rainbows appear in your room as the sun shines through brings an instant sense of wonder and awe to any environment.

Look at the Creativity area of your room and add small, whimsical touches, maybe a statue of a fairy or a four-leaf clover, or perhaps a childhood toy or a new creative project can occupy a special space. Bring in objects that remind you to be childlike and to have fun. In a more sophisticated setting, such as a professional office, use the Metal element in the form of statues, figurines, or furniture to enhance the energy of this area. Play with this wonderful energy of children and creativity and experience youth and energy returning to you daily.

Thirty-four

The Northwest: Helping People

The Northwest is the area in your environment that represents giving and receiving—helping people. It is the hospitality area and its energy promotes natural caring and kindness.

Environment

This area is the transition between the white of creativity and the black of career. Its color is gray, representing protection and mutual caring. A sharing of resources occurs here. The energy is related to commitment, pride, and dedication. Neither black nor white, there is room for flexibility and growth.

In our store, we have placed our hospitality feature in this area. We offer coffee, tea, water and other beverages to our customers. It represents a gesture of caring, of giving and receiving that enhances the energy of the entire store.

Look at the helping people area of your home or business now. What is there to remind you of sharing and caring? What attracts and benefits? What repels and limits? Notice for now what is there, and return at the end of this chapter to make your modifications.

Beliefs

The belief paradigm we work with in the Helping People area is the belief that if I give you something, then I have lost it versus the belief that giving opens me up to more receiving. It goes something like this: If I give you a smile or a hug, have I lost anything? Of course not. I have received a good feeling immediately in return. In fact, I had to have that good feeling before I gave it to you. If I did not have a smile, I could not have given it away. Now, what if I gave you something more material—let's say money. I give you ten dollars. Now you have my ten dollars and I apparently have it no more. But, I have opened myself up to receiving it back from another source. That's the notion of tithing. When I give freely, it is because I know that I have it to give. Knowing that I have it to give, I am opening up my energies to receiving it back and, as the Bible says, tenfold.

There is a catch. When I give with the feeling of sacrifice, I will receive sacrifice back. When I give with the feeling of abundance, I will receive abundance back. But do not look for it coming back necessarily from the same source. Giving and receiving is not indebtedness. It is not giving so someone will owe you something. I mentioned the coffee service in our store. We do not charge for coffee or tea. Some customers have some, look around the store, and make a purchase. But not always. Some folks enjoy the drink and leave. If giving is equal to losing, then we lost money on that person who left without buying. Right? Wrong! That person who left may go down the road and tell a friend about the hospitality and good feelings they experienced in the store. That friend may tell another person, and that person may look us up on the Web and make a purchase, or maybe not. It actually doesn't matter in the specifics. In order for us to give free drinks, we have to feel that we are abundant enough to provide them. By feeling that we are abundant, we attract abundance back to us.

The *Course in Miracles* states that giving and receiving are one. What we give, we receive, and what we receive we have given. That includes everything—attitudes, feelings, money, material objects—everything! We are giving and receiving all the time. When we give a smile, one comes back to us. When we give anger, it comes back to us. When we give money, it too comes back to us. We are teaching and learning by what we are giving and receiving.

Let this area of Helpful People be your focus for giving only that which you wish to receive. To receive love, give it. To receive money, give it. To receive peace, give it. What are you giving today?

Cures

The most notable cure for the area of Helping People is the use of mirrors. What we give to a mirror is reflected directly back to us. The mirror is a symbol for giving and receiving.

In Feng Shui, mirrors are used in two ways. First, they are used to reflect negativity away from an area. The eight-sided Baqua mirror is often hung on a door to reflect negative outside energy back before it is received inside. Traditionally, mirrors have been hung on doors that face cemeteries, power lines, traffic, negative neighbors, trash piles, and so on. This is so that what is given from the outside is not received into the home or office. In addition, mirrors are often used in apartment buildings to reflect the energies of your neighbors away. Placing a mirror face down on the floor will reflect the energy from below back down. The same is true when placing a mirror face up on the ceiling, to reflect energy upward. Mirrors placed on bathroom doors reflect energy away from "going down the drain."

Mirrors may also be used to reflect positive energies inside. If your window looks out onto a park, or trees, or a beautiful scene in nature, position a mirror so that the scene is reflected inside. Thus you receive beauty inside your home or office.

It is obvious that cures using mirrors are not directly related to helping people. In fact, they appear to be pushing people and objects away. Yet indirectly they do help. Negativity that is reflected back to its source will provide a lesson to the source. In the case of people, the more negativity a person gives out, the more they receive back, until they realize that there must be a better way. As we learn that the world is a reflection of our own thoughts and beliefs, we gain the power to change our world by changing what we are giving out. We look in the mirror and frown, and we receive a frown back. We look in the mirror and smile, and we receive a smile back. That is the lesson and it is really quite simple. It just takes practice to learn. Happy giving and receiving!

Thirty-five

The North: Career

The North is the your Career focus. Career represents your livelihood, line of business, and in some wonderful cases, your calling. When your career and your calling match, then you love what you are doing and what you are doing loves you!

Environment

Water is the element in the Career section. Water is formless and flowing. It conforms to and takes the shape of its container, yet seeks always to flow and expand. Water is the element that allows us to be in the flow and feel the energies that cycle through life. This flow of energy aids clarity and communication of our ideas into action.

Black is the color associated with the Career section of our environment. Black is the energy of absorption (black hole) and destruction of negative energy. It provides emotional protection and power. It is associated with money, career, experience, depth, and income.

Look now at the Career section of your home or office. What suggests flow and advancement there? What appears to be blocking your flow? What career ideas are present or absent there?

Beliefs

The basic paradigm here is work to earn a living versus work as vocation and calling. In the real world, most of us are heavily tied into the belief that we must work to earn money. We will pursue our calling only after we have worked long enough and hard enough to retire. Then we will do what we really want to do.

Many people become dissatisfied with their jobs and attempt to make what they love to do profitable. Some succeed, some fail. The difference between success and failure appears to lie in the core beliefs of the individual person. The best, and most risky, way to test your belief about job versus career is to pursue your dream. When you go for it, you will meet up directly with your fears. When you don't go for it, the universe will have a way to push you into your vocation, whether you want to go or not.

My husband and I had a plan. We are both physical therapists and planned to work at our respective jobs until we retired. Then we would pursue our calling to music and spiritual teaching and writing. Ten years ago we were both employed by large corporations and living in Augusta, Georgia. An Indian Swami (holy man) came to Augusta and we were invited to attend his concert. The spiritual energy of this man was tremendous. We spent a week with him, learning Kryia yoga and becoming spiritually energized. This was not something we actively sought out. We had at the time little interest in India, or holy men, or anything quite so esoteric.

The week after being with Swamiji, three things happened simultaneously. We visited the North Carolina mountains on vacation and through an accident of fate, met a realtor who took us on our current property. We walked on the land, knew that we were supposed to buy it, but did not have a clue as to how to pay for it or why we were buying it. Six weeks later we found ourselves closing on the land with no money down. The bank had put up 80 percent and the broker had put up the additional 20 percent. We returned to Augusta wondering what to do and received two phone calls. One was from a realtor who wanted to buy the property we owned at the time (it had not been on the market!), and the other was from a company who needed to hire two physical therapists for a hospital and home health agency ten miles from the land we had just purchased. The Universe was telling us something and we had to listen!

We moved to the mountains, still planning to work as physical therapists until we retired. That lasted about three years and then the Universe spoke again—in the form of being downsized from our jobs. At the same time, a small building on the major highway through the mountains became available for rent. The building was a half-mile from our home. We rented it and opened up a storefront and learning center. There seemed to be no other spiritual choice. We were being placed in the position that our job could become our calling.

The past five years have been spiritually, and economically, challenging. We have not, at this time, manifested the storybook ending of becoming rich and famous and financially independent. We have learned to love our jobs. We love getting up each morning and traveling the half-mile to our store. We love meeting our new and old customers in store and over the Internet. We love selecting our products based upon their energy of well being and love. We love seeing others love our selections.

We know that we are moving toward our vocations, our life callings. We cannot foresee what twists and bends in the river are ahead of us, but we are sure that each day we are flowing in the direction of our true purpose in this world. That is the meaning of career. Some people know what they are to do from birth and they just go and do it. Others, like us, stumble though all the old beliefs, clearing them one by one, until we finally reach the knowledge of who we are and what it is we are to do. Early retirement appears out of the picture financially just now, but, even if we could, we would not retire. The work we are doing now is meant to be done for the rest of our lives. That we know. We trust the flow to carry us through in our unexpected, but highly loved, new careers.

Cures

The most obvious Feng Shui cure for the Career area is use of the Water element. Water reminds up to flow with our lives, to allow the flow of career and money to come to us. The use of table fountains is the most common way to enhance the energy in your career section. Water features are visual reminders of the constant circulation and pooling of energy, as water travels from the fountain bowl, through the pump, and over the fountain. Water fountains can be enhanced with special designs that remind you of your vocation and career. Water flowing in your Career area allows you to grow and experiment in your job as you seek your vocation. And when you are in your vocation, it encourages the flow of money and abundance to come to you for your support.

Your fountain need not be elaborate. It only need have special meaning for you. Caring for your fountain, making sure it has plenty of water, running it at least a little while each day becomes a metaphor for the caring you are doing in your career. Allowing the fountain to represent the energy of your career reminds you that both are beautiful, flowing, and working properly.

So, look now at your Career area and find a place to add water. If you do not care for fountains, perhaps a small aquarium will do. If water is not appropriate to the area, how about a picture of water? Many Chinese restaurants have moving pictures of waterfalls or flowing rivers. I use to think that these electric pictures were flaky or tacky until I understood their meaning. They are allowing the energy of Water into an area. They remind the viewer of the power of water to move all obstacles in its path and find the perfect flow. May water move all obstacles in your career path until you find yourself in the perfect flow.

Thirty-six

The Northeast: Knowledge

The Northeast holds the energy of knowledge. This area is associated with two different types of knowing. The first consists of facts and ideas. The second is direct, nondualistic knowledge.

Environment

Water and Wood combine in this area of knowledge. The color is blue green—the colors of adventure and exploration combined with calming and relaxation. These colors of the sea and sky represent an openness to new ideas and insights.

This area of you home of business is a place for contemplation and learning. Use this area to explore new arenas of thought and act upon new perceptions.

Look at the Northeast area of your environment now. Is there a place for comfortable reading? What colors are now present? How inviting does this area feel in terms of learning? Are you ready to explore your mind and the minds of others here?

Beliefs

The balance of beliefs here is relying on facts versus trusting intuition. All facts have beliefs and feelings associated with them. All facts change. Long ago it was a fact that the world was flat. That fact contained the belief that if you traveled too far, you would simply fall off the world. The feelings attached to that fact was fear.

Another fact prevalent today is that the body is physical, made up of solid matter. The only reality is what can be viewed and measured. Because energy, like the wind, cannot be seen, it is not real. Holding onto the belief in only physical generates an amazing amount of fears and feelings of helplessness. If it is a fact that the body is a machine, and not influenced by the mind, then we are helpless victims to the fates of the machine. Yet another, new fact is emerging through quantum physics. The body is not solid, but vibrational. It is the vibration of quantum energy that forms the physical appearance of the body. Energy vibrations are influenced by the mind and emotions. This new fact leads to feelings of empowerment, and is based upon beliefs that we can influence our bodies. As author Louise Hay says, "You can heal your life."

Facts, with their thoughts and beliefs, are different than intuition or direct knowing. Nondualistic, choiceless awareness is associated with this type of knowledge. Some people know God. They don't just believe in God. They are not able to describe God in words. They simply know that God exists and is with them. This type of intuition or knowing guides our most profound actions. Examples abound of people who are driving down a familiar street and suddenly make an unexpected turn that appears illogical or not based on facts. Later they find out that if they had not made that turn, they would have been involved in a car accident or would have not discovered a new place to eat or relax. Following our intuition is equally as important as respecting the facts. Both must be in our lives.

Cures

Let the Knowledge area of your home or office represent both facts and intuition. Use this area for books, audio tapes, and inspirational posters. Design a quiet reading space here, accompanied by proper lighting and gentle music.

Along with your books, include a notepad or diary in which to record your ideas and insights. This is a good area to use when writing your business plan or personal mission statement.

Enlighten the area with the use of eight-sided Baqua mirrors. Allow the eight sides, plus the center, to bring you knowledge of the nine aspects of life. Expand your facts, give permission to your intuition, and find balance here.

Thirty-seven

The Center

The Center of your environment holds the energy of nurturing, balance, and stability. It provides the feeling of total support from the Universe and is the sum total of your choices.

Environment

Earth is the element associated with the Center. Earth represents grounding, steady progress, security, and caring. Earth is reliable, stable, solid, and confident. Earth endures endless change and still remains itself.

The color yellow is associated with the Center. Yellow represents longevity and acceptance of change through detachment. Yellow is a cheerful color. It opens and cleanses the mind and invites feelings of peaceful happiness and joyful bliss. Additional colors associated with the center are light yellow, beige, and tan.

Look now at the center of your home or room. Is there clutter, or is the space clear? Do the features seem stable and secure, or is there a sense of flightiness and instability? Is there anything in the center at all?

Beliefs

The balance in the center of our beliefs is between activity and stillness. Often when we are feeling "off center," our first tendency is to do something, anything, to fix the problem. There is an old adage that says: "When in worry, fear, or doubt; run in circles, scream, and shout." Activity gives us the illusion that something is being done. Because we are being active, surely the Universe will respond and help us. Unfortunately, frantic activity blocks the energy of the Universe. Thaddeus Golas, in his classic book *The Lazy Man's Guide to Enlightenment,* says that problems can never be resolved on the level at which they were created. To resolve problems, we must go higher. Going higher requires stillness. The ability to calm the mind through meditation is most crucial here. When the mind is calm and still, new insights emerge. New ways to solve old problems become apparent.

There is tremendous energy in stillness. Clearing the mind allows new beliefs to enter. Clearing the mind allows the energy of the universe to come into our lives. Just as the wind in autumn sweeps away fallen leaves, the energy of stillness sweeps away obstacles in our lives.

Cures

Make the center of your room a nurturing, healing space. If the Center is empty, add an area accent rug in earth tones. Arrange clay pots with rich potting soil and live plants in this area. Use square-shaped objects.

Long, flat rooflines enhance the stability of the center. Ceilings at angles are thought to create negative chi. Bamboo flutes, hung in pairs form the ceiling balance sharp angles or beams, deflecting negative energy and re-charging positive energy.

Small wind chimes, hung from the ceiling, will also enhance the peaceful energy of Earth. These chimes may sound in the breeze from ceiling fans, or air conditioning ducts. Use objects that remind you to be still and listen to the inner voice that always guides you to peace.

Thirty-eight

The Creative and Destructive Orders

The five elements in Feng Shui have creative and destructive orders in relationship to each other. The creative order follows the seasons and cycles of nature. The destructive order attempts to go against natural cycles. It is believed that using the elements in proper balance enhances one's fortune, while unbalance blocks good fortune. To provide a proper balance, first eliminate areas where the elements are being used in a destructive way, then combine elements according to the suggestions below.

Using the Elements in Combination

Wood is nourished by Water (water is necessary for wood to grow), and weakened by Metal (metal cuts wood). To improve health and family affairs, use fountains with growing plants. Contain water in resin or ceramic bowls rather than metal containers. Avoid using sharp, angular, metallic objects in the Health and Family area. Combining the colors green and black will enhance Wood energy. A black vase holding a lucky bamboo plant works well. Bonsai trees are most commonly seen in black bowls. Be creative with these two colors, using gentle black accents on green furniture, or black frames around photos or paintings of forests and trees. Let the growth of health be nourished by the Water element in your life.

The Fire of Fame and Success is weakened by Water (water extinguishes fire), and is nourished by Wood (wood provides fuel for fire to burn). To fan the fire of success in your environment, light candles safely contained in wood bases. Avoid placing candles too close to Water features. Combine the colors red and green to enhance success and fame—just like Christmas! Hang red tassels with green jade (called "Lucky Ties") to remind you of fame and fortune. Make a success poster using red and green lettering. Paint a picture, or find one, that uses vibrant red and green colors. Allow the energy of Health and Family to nourish fame and fortune in your life.

Earth is made by Fire and displaced by Wood. Candles in clay pots, bowls of sand and incense all enhance the centering and balance of Earth. Reds, pinks, and yellows are colors that energize Earth properties of balance, centering, and stillness. Have you ever noticed the colors of robes worn by Hindu and Buddhist monks? The robes are usually of silk or brilliant cotton and always combine shades of red, pink, orange, and yellow. That is a good example of the Fire element nourishing Earth. Try combining these colors in your own wardrobe and sense the difference. You will feel more stable, more grounded, and yet more vibrant when wearing these colors.

Metal is made by Earth and melted by Fire. To enhance creativity, combine earth and metal in sculptures, planters, and artistic creations. Using bright yellows and brilliant whites together spark the creative mind. Yellow "sticky" notes on white paper are often used in business to enhance creativity and new ideas.

Water is carried by Metal and stopped (dammed up) by Earth. To enhance career, flowing metal water sculptures are often placed outside of business buildings. Inside, even water fountains can bring the energy of Chi to one's career. The striking colors of black and white are also career boosters. Is it any wonder that for the past hundred years the classic business suit (for both men and women) has been black with a white shirt or blouse? Try placing abstract art in black and white on your walls. Energize your own thought by printing notes to yourself using big, place type, on white paper, of course.

Chi and the Elements

Chi is the expression of the energy force of life. Heaven Chi governs the celestial cycles; Earth Chi governs the ground. House Chi circulates through a dwelling and human Chi circulates through a person. The circulation of Chi without blockages, physical or mental, provides good fortune.

According to traditional Feng Shui, auspicious combinations of Chi include: 1) Chi plus Wood produces rain; 2) Chi plus Metal produces fine weather; 3) Chi plus Fire produces heat; 4) Chi plus Water produces cold; and 5) Chi plus Earth produces wind.

Chi nourishes our bodies, our hearts, and our minds. The Chinese practice of Chi Gong (*Chi* means "energy," *Gong* means "practice") is intended to circulate Chi within the body and to exchange Chi with the Universe. The more freely Chi circulates in our lives, the more success, prosperity, health, and harmony we experience. The secret to flow of this energy is in letting go. May you always let go and feel the flow.

Thirty-nine

The Reason for Energy SourceBook

Psychologist Abraham Maslow wrote that the big problems are: 1) To make the good person, the "responsible for himself and his own evolution" person; and 2) To make the good society—one species, one world.

To resolve the big problems is the reason for my writing this book and for you reading this book. To resolve these two problems is the reason for all study into spirituality, health, and healing. To resolve these two problems is, in fact, the reason that we are all here.

Abraham Maslow and the Hierarchy of Needs

You may remember Abraham Maslow, who in the in the late 1960s developed a hierarchical theory of human needs. Maslow was a humanistic psychologist, later a transpersonal psychologist, who believed that people are not controlled by mechanical forces alone. He focused on human potential, believing that humans strive to reach the highest levels of their capabilities. As a humanistic psychologist, Maslow is most recognized for his pyramid of needs. He investigated what motivates people. At the basic level, humans are motivated by biological and physiological needs: the need for oxygen, food, water—basic survival. Once these needs have been satisfied, the next motivation comes from security and safety needs: the need for shelter, clothing, a consistent daily lifestyle. Next are social needs: the need for love, affection, and belonging. Ego and self-esteem needs follow: the need for respect from others, to feel satisfied, self confident, and valuable. The top of Maslow's original pyramid was self-actualization and fulfillment needs: the need for work or vocation, the need to be involved in some cause beyond oneself.

Self-Transcendence

Prior to his death in 1970, Maslow was working on a final "need," that of self-transcendence. In studying self-actualized people, he found a unique group that had gone beyond the others in their development. This group was characterized by higher spiritual values and behaviors. In addition, this group reported more moments of "peak experiences" happening in their daily lives. Peak experiences have certain basic characteristics that include: a giving up of the past and future; an innocence of perceiving and behaving, a connection to the Real Self through the loss of ego and self-forgetfulness; strength and courage; acceptance and a positive attitude, spontaneity, and expressiveness; integration of Being values; and trust.

These characteristics are found in people who experience source energy through meditation and other activities described in this book. Only by going beyond one's self can one discover the ultimate Self that is Source.

Maslow went on to list the behaviors he discovered that lead toward peak experiences and a spiritual way of Being in the world.

Behaviors leading towards self-transcendence include:

- Experiencing fully, vividly, selflessly with full concentration and total absorption.
- Making growth-choices instead of fear choices.
- Understanding that there is a self to be actualized and listening to the impulse voices within to let the self emerge.
- When in doubt, being honest.

- Choosing wisely by listening to own self at each moment in life.
- Using one's intelligence—working to do well the thing one wants to do.
- Inviting peak experiences to occur in one's life.
- Opening oneself up to oneself and making oneself "sacred under the aspect of eternity."

Being Values

Maslow concluded that there are fourteen ultimate values—"Being Values"—that enable the problems of the individual and the world to be resolved. These values include: Truth (honesty); Goodness (benevolence); Beauty (rightness); Wholeness (interconnectedness); Aliveness (spontaneity); Uniqueness (individuality); Perfection (nothing lacking); Completion (fulfillment); Justice (fairness); Simplicity (essentiality); Richness (nothing is unimportant); Effortlessness (ease and lack of strain); Playfulness (humor and fun); and Self-sufficiency (not needing anything other than itself in order to be itself).

Being Values are the characteristics of being fully human, the preferences of full human people, the characteristics of selfhood or identity in peak experiences. They are characteristic of ideal art, ideal children, ideal theories, ideal science and knowledge. They are the far goals of all psychotherapies, the far goals of all education, the far goals of religions. They are the characteristics of the ideally good environment and of the ideally good society.

Energy SourceBook

I believe the ultimate reason to experience source energy is to create the good person, the good society, and the good world. To go inside the self, to explore the self, and finally to transcend the self in service of good.

Imagine a world of self-transcendent beings. Imagine every store you shop at, every company representative you deal with, every person in every car on every highway, and every family member demonstrating the Being Values. Hard to picture? That's okay. Because we will all be there one day. It is a basic need of every individual. And every person works in his or her own way to try and fulfill that need. That's why we are here on the earth plane. That is what our Souls are guiding us toward. So begin the journey within yourself. Feel the energy flowing through you; practice daily; and watch miracles unfold in your life.

This book ends with a "Loving Kindness Meditation." Notice that the meditation begins with "I," then proceeds to "You," and finally expands to "All." We change the world by changing ourselves. That is the only way the world changes. Happy journeys, dear reader! Thank you for traveling this path with me at this time. May you be *well.*

Loving Kindness Meditation

May I be filled with loving kindness.
May I be Well.
May I be peaceful and at ease.
May I be Happy.
May You be filled with loving kindness.
May You be Well.
May You be peaceful and at ease.
May You be Happy.
May All Beings be filled with loving kindness.
May All Beings be Well.
May All Beings be peaceful and at ease.
May All Beings be Happy.
And So it Is!

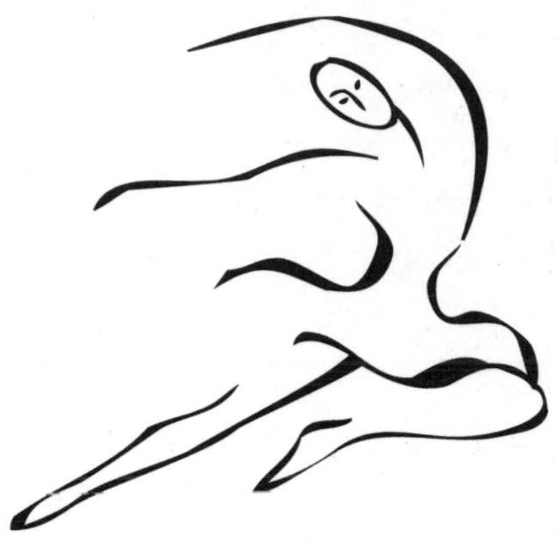

References and Resources

Glossary

Breathing: refers to specific activities that involve the breath in order to access deeper states of relaxation and meditation.

Chakra: an ancient Sanskrit term for "spinning wheel of energy." There are numerous chakra locations within the physical body, places where energy infuses mind and matter. This book explores the seven major chakra centers.

Chi Energy: the word *Chi* literally means "energy." This unseen energy circulates through and around the body as well as through and around the universe. Mastery of Chi energy provides strength, health, and healing.

Color: the vibrations of different colors are essential to physical and mental well being. Colors are explored using the chakra system as well as the Feng Shui system of color management and enhancement.

Direction: in many traditions, the direction of a home or room or bed represents significant attributes and abilities. This book explores the directions according to Feng Shui tradition. The attributes of these directions overlap with Native American lore, but are not the same in every case.

"Dis-ease": while the term disease refers to a set of signs and symptoms, dis-ease refers to a lack of ease in the body's energy system. This lack of ease can be brought into ease and balance through energy work, meditation, relaxation, nutrition, and a variety of means described in this book.

Elements: refers to the characteristics and nature of the basic elements seen on earth with reference to Polarity Therapy and Feng Shui. Elements in most cases represent the qualities of energy flowing through the body or through an environment. Polarity elements include: Ether, Air, Fire, Water, and Earth; while Feng Shui elements add Metal and Wood to Water, Fire and Earth.

Emotions: basic emotions governing our happiness, or lack there of, are discussed in relation to chakras and energies.

Exercises: throughout this book, simple exercises and activities are offered to complement the information provided and bring about greater states of well being.

Feng Shui: literally means "wind and water," and is defined as the art and science of arranging objects in a room or environment to enhance the flow of Chi (energy) to bring about health, success, and prosperity.

Feng Shui Cure: refers to a specific object placed in an environment to enhance the flow of Chi. Cures include crystals, flutes, chimes, and more.

Issues: refers to the basic life tasks every person works on at one point of another in their lives. Common issues include health, wealth, and relationships.

Meditation: is a tool for going inside and directing the mind to find peace and contentment. It is a skill that can be developed by anyone, and used to enhance life.

Nutrition: refers to basic foods that may be eaten to balance energy flows in the body, thus improving mental and physical health.

Planes of Consciousness: are the mental states one may access through deep relaxation and meditation.

Relaxation: is a skill little developed in today's population, yet is responsible for changing the body from a state of dis-ease, to a state of ease and well being.

Stress: is a state of body dis-ease, brought about by mental factors and the inability to direct the mind through meditation.

Annotated Bibliography

Section One

Anonymous (1975). *A Course in Miracles.* Foundation for Inner Peace, Mill Valley, CA.

A spiritual study of love and forgiveness through extensive text and 365 workbook lessons.

Anderson, U.S. (1954). *Three Magic Words.* Melvin Powers Wilshire Book Company, Hollywood, CA.

The first metaphysical book we read—it changed our lives!

Allen, James (1991). *As I Think.* DeVorss Publications, Marina del Rey, CA.

Every sentence in this book in as affirmation.

Benson, Herbert, M.D. (1975). *The Relaxation Response.* Avon Books, NY.

A generic guide to Western mantra meditation research and practice.

———. (1984). *Beyond the Relaxation Response.* Avon Books, NY.

Further resources on Western mantra meditation.

Capra, F. (1982). *The Turning Point: Science, Society, and the Rising Culture.* New York: Bantam Books.

An great overview of science and philosophy of changing paradigms and belief systems in society.

Carrington (1984) in Woolfolk & Lehrer. *Principles and Practice of Stress Management.* Guilford Press, New York.

Comprehensive guide to research and practice of relaxation and meditation.

Chan, Luke (1999). *101 Miracles of Natural Healing.* Benefactor Press, West Chester, OH.

Describes the Basic Forms and Results of Chi-Lel Chi Gong.

Dass, Ram (1978, 1990). *Journey of Awakening—A Meditator's Guide.* Bantam Books, New York.

Excellent overview of meditation techniques!

Deepak Chopra, M.D. *Ageless Body, Timeless Mind, Unconditional Life, Wisdom Within.*

Any book by Dr. Chopra will lead you to vast insights and paradigm shifts, change and healing.

Epstein, Gerald, MD (1989) *Healing Visualizations: Creating Health Through Imagery.* Bantam Books, New York.

Wonderful, quick, healing affirmations for illness and disease.

Ferguson, M. (1980). *The Aquarian Conspiracy: Personal and Social Transformation in the 1980s.* Los Angeles: J. P. Tarcher, Inc.

A classic book on changing beliefs, worldviews and paradigms.

Gass, Robert. *On Wings of Song—Songs of Healing* CD. Spring Hill Music, Boulder, Co.

Mantras in English.Check out his complete collection!

Goldman, Jonathan. *Chakra Chants*—CD from Etherean Music.

Seven tracks of sound and mantras for Chakra Balancing

Grabhorn, Lynn (2000). *Excuse Me, Your Life is Waiting.* Hampton Roads Publishing, Charlottesville, VA.

Practical and delightful book on using feelings to turn wants and desires into actual experience.

Hay, Louise (1984, 1987). *You Can Heal Your Life.* Hay House, Carlsbad, CA.

Overall best "beginner" book for changing your life!

Johnson, Willard (1982) *Riding the Ox Home: A History of Meditation from Shamanism to Science.* Beacon Press, Boston.

Classic book about meditation and meaning.

Kabat-Zinn, Jon. *Full Catastrophe Living: Using the Wisdom of Your Body and Mind to Face Stress/Pain/Illness. Wherever You Go, There You Are: Mindfulness Meditation in Everyday Life.*

Excellent books on the practice of mindfulness meditation.

Kaur, Singh and Kim Robertson. *Crimson Collection* CDs. Invincible Productions, Phoenix, AZ.

Six different mantras for different purposes. Great listening!

Konicov, Barrie (1978). Potentials Unlimited, Inc. 4808-H Broadmoor, SE. Grand Rapids, MI 49508.

Self-hypnosis tapes for powerful change.

Lansdowne, Zachary (1986). *Chakras and Esoteric Healing.*

Great book on exploring hierarchies and energy development.

Levine, Stephen (1979, 1989). *A Gradual Awakening.* Anchor Books, New York.

The best layman's book to meditation on the market!

Murphy, Joseph (1963, 2000). *The Power of Your Subconscious Mind.* Bantam Books, New York.

Practical exploration and guide to changing your subconscious beliefs and affirming your desires.

Price, John Randolph (1987). *The Abundance Book.* Hay House, Carlsbad, CA.

A 40-day plan for change using 10 powerful affirmations.

Vaughan, F. (1986). *The Inward Arc: Healing and Wholeness in Psychotherapy and Spirituality.* Boston: New Science Library, Shambhala.

Great theoretical overview of adult psychology and development.

Yutang, L., translator (1948). *The Wisdom of Lao Tse.* Random House, New York.

The best and most complete translation of the classic Tao.

Zemach-Bersin, David. *Relaxercise: The Easy Way to Health and Fitness.* HR 0-06-250992-6.

Great exercise book for gentle, relaxing activity.

Section Two

Brennan, Barbara (1987). *Hands of Light.* Bantam Books, New York.

In-depth study of chakra energy and healing techniques.

Brennan, Barbara (1993). *Light Emerging.* Bantam Books, New York.

Continuation of her first book, with emphasis on self-healing.

Garner-Gordon, Joy (1988). *Color and Crystals: A Journey Through the Chakras.* Crossing Press, Freedom, CA.

Nice review of chakras, gemstones, archetypes, and more.

Hay, Louise and Joshua Leeds (1986). *Songs of Affirmation: Chants and Meditations.* Hay House, Santa Monica, CA.

Excellent cassette of healing chants and meditations.

Henry, Jill and Charles Henry (1990). *10-Minute Rainbow Tune-Up Tape.* Resources for Well Being, Martinez, GA (available through www.mountainvalleycenter.com).

Jones, Alex (1982). *Seven Mansions of Color.* DeVorss & Co. Marina del Rey, CA.

Esoteric document on chakras and the seven rays of color.

Jones, Laurie Beth (1996). *The Path: Creating Your Mission Statement for Work and for Life.* Hyperion, New York, NY.

Wonderful guidelines and examples for creating your own mission statement.

Myss, Caroline (1996). *Anatomy of Spirit.* Crown Publishers, Random House, New York.

Uses the metaphor of chakras to explore archetypal body/mind types and healing.

Nadequ, Roland and Deborah Riegel (1994). *I Am Worthy.* Audio tape. I Am Worthy, Inc. Austin, TX.

Great affirmations to heal and awaken love and success.

Paulson, Genevieve (1991). *Kundalini and the Chakras.* Llewellyn Publications, St. Paul, MN.

Fun book with lots of exercises for chakra work.

Rendel, Peter (1979). *Understanding the Chakras.* Harper/Collins, London.

Ruskin, John(2000). *Emotional Clearing.* Broadway Books, a division of Random House, New York, NY (Originally published by R. Wyler and Company).

Classic information about the chakras.

Sharamon, Shalila and Bodo Baginski (1991). *The Chakra Handbook.* Federal Republic of Germany.

Good, concise chakra information.

Vaughn, Frances (1985). *The Inward Arc.* New Science Library, Boston, MA.

Wonderful examination of psychology and spirituality.

Section Three

American Polarity Therapy Association (www.polaritytherapy.org) can be contacted at P. O. Box 19858, Boulder, CO 80308.

Beaulieu, John (1994). *Polarity Therapy Workbook.* Biosonic Enterprises, New York.

Comprehensive treatment guide using polarity therapy techniques.

Campbell, Morag (1995) *Quinta Essentia.* The Five Elements Masterworks, Devon, England.

Wonderful descriptions of the five elements in Polarity Therapy.

Chitty, John and Mary Louise Muller (1990). *Energy Exercises: Easy Exercises for Health and Vitality.* Polarity Press, Boulder, CO.

Great, simple, abundant exercises for balancing body energies. Each exercise is referenced to the five elements.

Seidman, Maruti (1999). *A Guide to Polarity Therapy: The Gentle Art of Hands-on Healing.* North Atlantic Books, Berkeley, CA.

Good overview of Polarity Therapy.

Stone, Randolph, DC, DO (1985). *Health Building: The Conscious Art of Living Well.* CRCS Wellness Books, Summertown, TN.

A layperson's book from the Source of Polarity Therapy.

——. (1986). *Polarity Therapy Volume One: The Complete Collected Works.* CRCS Publications, Sebastopol, CA.

Dr. Stone's original works, diagrams, and explanations of Polarity Therapy.

——. (1987). *Polarity Therapy, Volume Two: The Complete Collected Works.* CRCS Publications, Sebastopol, CA.

A continuation of Dr. Stone's notes.

Young, Phil (1990). *The Art of Polarity Therapy: A Practitioner's Perspective.* Prism Press, Dorsett, UK.

Good overview of Polarity Therapy.

Special thanks to my Polarity teacher, Angela Plum, Ph.D., RPP, Academy of Natural Therapies, Marshall, NC.

Section Four

Anonymous (1975). Foundation for Inner Peace, Mill Valley, CA.

A spiritual self-study guide for letting go of the ego and finding the Spirit of Love

Collins, Terah Kathryn (1996). *The Western Guide to Feng Shui.* Hay House, Carlsbad, CA.

Great starter book for re-arranging your home or office.

Finster, Elaine Jay (1991–1999). *Health, Wealth, and Balance Through Feng Shui.* New Age Concepts, Bailey, CO.

Good description of different schools of Feng Shui and basic elements.

Freeman, James Sillet (1978). *The Story of Unity.* Unity Books, Unity Village, Missouri.

The story of the founders of the Unity Church.

Grabhorn, Lynn (2000). *Excuse Me, Your Life Is Waiting.* Hampton Roads Publishing, Charlottesville, VA.

Practical and delightful book on using feelings to turn wants and desires into actual experience.

Fretwell, Sally (2000–2001). *Feng Shui: Back to Balance.* New World Library: Novato, CA.

Great descriptions of the elements, colors, and meanings in Feng Shui.

Golas, Thaddeus (1972). *The Lazy Man's Guide to Enlightenment.* New York: Bantam Books.

Simple, profound, book about going higher and happier.

Lau, Kwan (1996). *Feng Shui for Today.* Tengu Books, Trumbull, CT.

Concise overview into compass directions and meanings in arranging a home or room.

Chapter 39: The Reason for Energy SourceBook

Henry, Jill N. (1988). *Development and Learning for Transformation: A Model Linking Lifelong Learning and Transpersonal Psychology.* Doctoral Dissertation, University of Georgia, Athens, GA.

Original studies of transformation and change by the author.

Maslow, Abraham H. (1964). *Religion, Values and Peak Experiences.* Ohio State University Press, Columbus, Ohio.

Maslow's experience with peak meditative experiences.

——. (1968). *Toward a Psychology of Being.* D. Van Nostrand Company, 1968.

Maslow's basic hierarchy of needs.

——. (1969). "The Farther Reaches of Human Nature," *Journal of Transpersonal Psychology.* 1 (1), 1–9.

——. (1969b). "Various Meaning of Transcendence," *Journal of Transpersonal Psychology.* 1 (1), 56–66.

——. (1969c). "Theory Z," *Journal of Transpersonal Psychology.* 1 (2), 31–47.

Maslow helped create the Journal of Transpersonal Psychology and was one of its first authors.

Other Classic Books and Resources for Further Study

Allen, Marc, ed. (1987). *As You Think,* by James Allen. San Rafael, CA: Whatever Publishing, Inc.

Anderson, U. S. (1954). *Three Magic Words.* No. Hollywood, CA: Melvin Powers/Wilshire Book Company.

Bach, Richard (1977). *Illusions: The Adventures of a Reluctant Messiah.* New York: Dell Publishing Co.

Bucke, Richard Maurice M.D. (1901). *Cosmic Consciousness.* Paperback edition, 1969, New York, NY: E. P. Dutton.

Bynner, Witter. (1972). *The Way of Life According to Lao Tzu.* New York: Perigee Book.

Cady, Emile (Nd). *Lessons in Truth.* Unity Village, Missouri: Unity Books.

Capra, Fritjof (1983). *The Turning Point: Science, Society, and the Rising Culture.* New York: Bantam Books.

Carlson,Richard and Benjamin Shield, eds. *Healers on Healing.* Los Angeles: Jeremy P. Tarcher, Inc.

Custer, Dan (1960). *The Miracle of Mind Power.* Englewood Cliffs, NJ: Prentice Hall, Inc.

Dass, Ram (1978). *Journey of Awakening: A Meditator's Guidebook.* New York: Bantam Books.

Fox, Emmet (1946). *Make Your Life Worthwhile.* San Francisco: Harper & Row.

Ferguson,Marilyn (1980). *The Aquarian Conspiracy: Personal and Social Transformation in the 1980s.* Los Angeles: J. P. Tarcher, Inc.

Gawain, Shakti (1982). *Creative Visualization.* New York, NY: Bantam Books.

Golas, Thaddeus (1972). *The Lazy Man's Guide to Enlightenment.* New York, NY: Bantam Books.

Hay, Louise (1984). *You Can Heal Your Life.* Carson, CA: Hay House, Inc.

Holmes, Ernest (1957). *The Basic Ideas of Science of Mind.* Los Angeles, CA: Science of Mind Publications.

Jampolsky, Gerald G. M.D. (1970). *Love Is Letting Go of Fear.* New York: Bantam Books.

Krishnamurti, J. (1964). *Think on These Things.* New York, NY: Harper & Row.

Levine, Stephen (1979). *A Gradual Awakening.* New York, NY: Anchor Books.

Lilly, John M. D. (1972). *The Center of the Cyclone: An Autobiography of Inner Space.* New York, NY: Julian Press.

Locke, Steven, M. D. and Douglas Colligan (1986). *Healer Within.* New York, NY: New American Library Mentor book.

Maslow, A. H. (1971). *The Farther Reaches of Human Nature.* New York, NY: Viking Press.

Ponder, Catherine (1985). *The Dynamic Laws of Healing.* Marina del Rey, CA: DeVorss & Company.

Price, John R. (1985). *Practical Spirituality.* Boerne, Texas: Quartus Books.

Progoff, Ira (1980). *The Practice of Process Meditation.* New York, NY: Dialogue House Library.

Rengel, Peter. (1987). *Seeds of Light: Inspriations From My Higher Self.* Tiburon, CA: H. J. Kramer.

Rodegast, Pat, and Judith Stanton (1885). *Emmanuel's Book: A Manual for Living Comfortably in the Cosmos.* New York, NY: Bantam Books.

Roman, Sanaya and Duane Parker (1988). *Creating Money: Keys to Abundance.* Tilburon, CA: H. J. Kramer, Inc.

Silva, J. and P. Miele (1977). *The Silva Mind Control Method.* New York, NY: Simon & Schuster, Inc.

Small, Jacquelyn (1982). *Transformers: The Therapists of the Future.* Marina del Rey, CA: DeVorss & Company.

Smith, Harry Douglas (1965). *The Secret of Instantaneous Healing.* New York, NY: Parker Publishing Company, Inc.

Smith, Huston (1958). *The Religions of Man.* New York, NY: Harper & Row.

Tart, C., ed. (1983). *Transpersonal Psychologies.* El Cerrito, CA: Psychological Processes, Inc. (originally published in 1975 by Harper & Row).

Trungpa, Chogyam (1973). *Cutting Through Spiritual Materialism.* Boston: Shambhala.

Vaughan, Frances (1986). *The Inward Arc: Healing and Wholeness in Psychotherapy and Spirituality.* Boston: New Science Library, Shambhala.

Watts, Alan W. (1951). *The Wisdom of Insecurity: A Message for an Age of Anxiety.* New York, NY: Vintage Books.

Wilber, Ken (1977). *Spectrum of Consciousness.* Wheaton, IL: Theosophical Publishing House.

——. (1981). *No Boundary: Eastern and Western Approaches to Personal Growth.* Boston: New Science Library, Shambhala.

——. (1986). *Up from Eden: A Transpersonal View of Human Evolution.* Boston: New Science Library, Shambhala.

Williams, Paul (1987). *Remember Your Essence.* New York, NY: Harmony Books.

Wing, R. L. (1986). *The Tao of Power.* New York, NY: Dophin Books/Doubleday and Company.

Yutang, Lin (1948). *The Wisdom of Lao Tse.* New York, NY: Random House, Inc.

Index